HUMAN BODY HOW IT WORKS?

YUNUS EMRE PEKCICI

ISBN: 9798648098060
E-ISBN: 9786254001031

~ Contents ~

Introduction: Understanding Key of the Book

Body is a mechanism which is working in order. That order has got four philosophies. Balance, Effect, Reflect, Adaptation. These are the keys to understand every temporary or permanent changes in the body. Every title in this book, explaining different changes in the body which directly affect our health, activity performance and appearance.

There is always an accepted balance in the body. An effect comes through body and gets a reflect. An effect always gets a reflect. If that effect insists on coming through; that reflection will give its own place to adaptation. Adaptation takes the place and changes the "accepted balance" in order to not give reflects anymore. Because accepting new situation is easier and more acceptable in order to fit survival mentality, which is the mentality of the human body.

1) Balance:

Balance is the normal form of the body; "normal" term depends for everybody. The balance rules apply to every cell; therefore, to every organ in the body. Heart, lungs, muscles, nerves and activity form of theirs. Balance is not a fixed rule. "The Balance" may change with constant adaptations and find another form but the name would be still "The Balance". Changing balance is not that easy but not that hard as well.

2) Effect:

Every action to the body from the inside and outside is an effect. Eating food is an outside effect. The ingredients of food or drink effecting body. Creating a hormone in the body, is an inside effect or giving the stimulation of moving to a muscle is an inside effect. Those effects created by body itself and becoming a reason of starting a reflect.

3) Reflect:

Reflect is always bounded to an effect. Almost everything we know as a verb is an effect for the body. Against those effects body always has got an answer. If body get punched by somebody else, it is an effect; creating pain and supportive reflexes are reflects to that effect.

Body creates a hormone which is "gonadotropin releasing hormone", it is an effect. The reflect to that, is creating a chain of actions which is known as entering puberty.

Every action in the body is happening according to an effect and reflect.

4) Adaptation:

Adaptation is the name of creating "The New Balance". After continues effects and reflects body gets adapted to situation. Putting itself in a form which is giving less reflects to same effects. If a person continues to get punched by somebody else, eventually the pain he is feeling and the fear body getting into will be lower. Boxers get durable to being punched, and more durable compared to normal people.

Adaptation happens both physically and mentally. We get used to everything.

Adaptation is the fourth and end key of the process. And a key of survival of human. Human adaptation makes him stronger against nature and himself.

Improvements, developments we name them. That

is a form of adaptation which occurs with; constantly applying same effect-reflect chain; which is challenging body limits. Carrying weights and weightlifting is a perfect example to this. Lifting challenging weights in the same way for every day, eventually brings the ability of lifting heavier weights or lifting same weights much faster.

However; body does not always make improvement or development; body also adapts in opposite way. Gets weaker, loses muscle, gets aged… So, is it evolution or revolution, may be devolution?

Chapter 1:

Hardware of Movement and Usage of Them

It Is Not Evolution, It Is Revolution

As a human being; we are thinking that, we have to make progress. Get much more strength, get much more muscle mass, get much more balance etc. These are improvements for us, but are these really?

Brain is a vital organ which tries to keep our bodies in "optimum range" according to our lifestyle. Brain doesn't have its own emotions or decisions. We are the one who is deciding; the soul, the energy or whatever you call. Brain is just adapted to do decisions and actions.

Explanation with an example; when a bacteria kind enters your body, your brain sends white blood cells to that area; also, to make them work more efficient, makes your body heat higher, and creates inflammation areas to fight and reconstruct in it. When you hear in this way, you would say "Yes, it is a nice method". But on the outside, you are freezing due to your body heat, you can't swallow due to throat inflammation, and you feel weak and unable to move because of ongoing fight inside of your body.

Brain just adapted to situation and trying to bring and keep your life to "optimum range", by damaging your feels for a while.

With every action of brain, there has to be reason behind of that. If your metabolism getting faster or your cells are growing, or you get inflammation in your joints, or whatever you are into; brain isn't deciding anything. It always reflects to the causation. While trying to achieve something good which is desired such as beautiful body; we are trying to create a causation, or we are trying to clear away another causation. Along with, this causation change; brain does its job which is all metabolic actions, which we know as physiology.

Sometimes these causations are external factors and sometimes internal factors. Example, for internal factor; entering puberty, starting along with morphologic and hormonal changing period. Our body designed to release "gonadotropin-releasing hormone" in the specific time which is coded in our DNA. So, this hormone; releases gonadotropin, then gonadotropin starts to flow in your blood. The related fields in our brain or other hormone releasing organs; detect it and release or stop to release some other hormones. There are many changes becoming in content of blood in the terms of hormone. Each cell only detects the one hormone which is related to that via specialized receptors to that hormone. After detecting the hormone, cell starts to create changes which is coded in its DNA so in its own brain.

This was an example of an internal causation and reaction chain of the brain and body. If we go back to the beginning of the cycle, to gonadotropin releasing hormone. Humans could create this hormone by some methods in laboratory. We could inject this hormone into blood or directly to the field in the body. Afterwards puberty like situation starts again with the effect of hormone. But in this example, subject became an external causation. However, it is not a supported method; except some special illness situations. Because you wouldn't want to mess with regular cycle of internal causations, which will be explained in upcoming topics.

Sometimes these causations are natural external factors. And most common one is eating food. Every vitamin, mineral, protein, carb etc. has different effect in our bodies. And they start a reaction chain. For example; when you take caffeine to your body, as a result your metabolism starts to work faster. Because you have manipulated your body with external causation.

Your body doesn't think caffeine is a good thing or bad thing. You are the one who is thinking in this way.

Your body is a machine. Like a vending machine, if you send a coin through inside, machine will start and give the result. But you have got thousands of vending machines in your body. Each action is required another kind of coin. But all the focus point on this "Vending machine doesn't care about your wishes or requests, they only care coins". In the terms of improvement and development; we have to put right coin to start the mechanism to get results which we want.

The main reason of this much explanation is to understand whole improvement and development system of body. Subject may be sport, medicine, life quality, health so on. No matter which subject it is, there is always a direct or undirect relation with muscles in the body. Along with the creation of movement and so our meaning of "living creature", they are also the main part of metabolism. Every other organ in the body stands in there just for two organs in the body. Brain and muscle.

Understanding reactional changes in the muscles with workout and activity types, will increase your vision and knowledge about designing a workout, a treatment and a lifestyle program. These designing improvement is the main subject of increasing the life quality, health quality, sportive activity quality. Even for most of treatments which are occurred with internal causation; are related with skeletal muscles in the body. Understanding its physiology is the key to understand how to treat and work them.

Science of causations and reactions: Physiology. Physiology of human body will be explained but we are starting with motor and movement power of the body: Muscle.

Physiology of The Muscle:

Humans are born with organs, some of them doesn't get multiplied in cellular base. For example, neuron cells, doesn't make mitosis and multiplies, only get mass. In muscle side, number of muscle fibers are designed before we are born. No one cannot increase number of fibers. but everyone could enlarge or make smaller their muscle cells, henceforth fiber's size and power.

Every human has got skeletal muscle mostly in same anatomic design. Starting and ending points etc. 320 pairs of muscles are placed in our bodies. Each muscle has got 10 to 100 fibers in it. Those fibers are easily could be seen by eye if you take over the skin. Those are single cells which includes many components inside of them. Most importantly "Sarcomere" "Nucleus" and "Mitochondria" which are more than one in a single fiber.

Duty of nucleus is managing the cell. How much the cell gets bigger, that much the nucleus multiplies. You need many more manager for bigger companies.

Primer function of mitochondria is providing energy to the cell via its dissolve protocol. By using oxygen and glucose. In the presence of enough oxygen in the cell there is aerobic fermentation happening and that brings us significant amount of ATP which is energy for us. So, the idea is how much you need to spend energy in the presence of oxygen in the cell that much mitochondria are required.

Actually, the functions of organelles those are said, mostly explains what we should do to improve or not. Yet, a longer explanation is always better. However, before we understand the cellular changes, we have to understand the types of fibers first. Because people have got 3 kind of fibers which all shows different physiological and functional specialty.

A sportsman, a trainer, a doctor or a normal person who want to make a body; healthier or stronger or faster must know these fiber types. Because each one of them stands for different purpose in a different kind of working protocol. Learning that protocol gives us the information of how to make activities and how to eat our nutrition in order to improve, develop functions of the body or treat illnesses such as diabetics or not to get them in the first place.

Fiber Types:

There are 3 different type of fibers commonly exist in human body. We are not talking about exceptions. Which are type I, type IIa, type IIb.

Each one of them are serving to different purposes with different ingredient of theirs.

In the philosophy of body, there is one rule. Adaptation hence revolution.

In the means of the revolution; you can't keep two ideology at the same time. Also, you can't keep the previous idea with the new idea. So, brain chooses the dominant on the behalf of causations. In the muscle fibers it is; choosing having type 1 or type 2. In other words, to be stronger or be enduring. There is always a choose, no exception. These both cannot be together at the same time. Many things on the body is going according to same ideology. You can't have the day and the night at the same time. But there are mixing points, like mid-afternoon or sunrise. So, there are always type1 and type 2a and 2b fibers in everyone. But percentage of these changes. Henceforth, you could choose to be much closer to the day or to be much closer to the night. Stronger or enduring.

Many differences occur due to causation changes; but changes in the terms of nucleus and mitochondria are the most important for us. Their change is primer effect on fiber type changing.

Changing of Types

 * In the brain perspective: "This human trying to use excessive force on its muscle; and you, components of that muscle, get stronger; by getting bigger. Adapt to the situation. "Nucleus numbers increase in order to provide getting bigger of cell. And nucleus numbers increase since the cell needs to get big. It has been told to them, by brain with hormones and stimulations.

 * In the brain perspective: "This human trying to use its muscle for long periods, forcing it's oxidative energy limits. And components of that muscle, get enduring, by getting smaller and creating much more energy in long term, get yourself into saving mode. "Nucleus number decreases in order to provide getting smaller of cell. And nucleus number decreases cell needs to get small. Also, mitochondria number increases in order to create more ATP in the long term with much more efficient way which is oxidative fermentation. It has been told to them, by brain with hormones and stimulations.

A person could think that; "But while running marathon or etc. which is longer and easier compared to 6 reps of jumping squats or heavy weight squat when considered in the unit of time. Because you are using much more ATP in unit of time while making jumping squats or any other heavy weight activity."

Actually, this idea is right, but there are other two mechanism for short term muscle contraction energy source. Which are glycogen and ATP-Creatine Phosphate source. It provides many ATP to the cell in unit of time for a short term which makes this action possible. If you cannot refill your ATP-CP source or glycoses source or it is already empty you will not be able to create any force. Simply your body won't move in a way that makes heavy weight liftings or jump squats, even you have enough muscle mass for that.

While running marathon, your body will keep continue to run; because it is always providing enough oxygen to the mitochondria. But when the creation of ATP Is not enough to run, you would still run but your body would stop to create ATP for other organs such as brain to keep enough oxygen in your legs. Which is the main reason; why marathon runners are gone into shock after race or during race, and they can't respond your answers, or they just fade away. Sometimes consciousness comes after long running; due to, running is a reflex movement but consciousness not. And body's priority is reflex movements. Which is designed to keep us alive. Heart beating, breathing, and if you are marathon runner, it is running; because body is thinking in survival way. So, body is canalizing current ATP sources and ATP creation to the more necessary survival activities instead of internal organs. With an exception running is gained after born reflex. One who never run, will not have this reflex and will not put into priority.

And another idea: "Why the cells are getting smaller while turning into another type. We want bigger cells; due to have bigger muscles. Big muscles look good."

As It is mentioned before; brain doesn't think in emotional way, it is us who thinks in this way. So, brain makes cells smaller in order to spend less energy. Because contraction of a big cell which is fiber, requires much more energy. If a person is using them for long time, brain is going through saving mode, and makes cells smaller. And in the first place they don't need to be big, aren't they? That human is not using them to create force in frequently. May he jump twice a day or using ladders instead of elevator which requires bigger muscle cells; but that is not enough causation to prevent that change completely. Because that person is walking for 2 hours in a day already. One causation is so frequent which may cover the other. Which is dominant that wins. But as It is mentioned, there is a mixing point. This changing never happens as %100 percent. Even in a marathon runner there still would be around of %30 strength fibers even though not using them at all in anytime. In a power weightlifter there would be still around of %30-40 endurance fibers. This topic will be understood better after reading specifications of the types.

There is no evolution, there is always a change, so revolution. But what if someone who never uses its muscles, may be someone in coma or on computer all day long or someone getting aged. What happens then, could we say there is still a changing? What about nucleuses, mitochondria etc. Explanation is; there is no evolution or revolution at there but there is devolution.

"If we are not using them, why we need them at all" – Brain (Since Born)

They still using energy and brain thinking about survival, always. The human is not using his muscles for a long term, those muscle using energy unnecessarily even while not using, because of basal metabolism. Why brain should keep that tap open which empties the pool. It simply tries to close if you insist on that lifestyle.

Even a person is not insisting on inactivity, body still is going to take muscles and strength away from that person with the age. There is no known causation for that, it is just coded in DNA like puberty, which we don't have puissance on it. That is why people cannot find a cure to aging because there is no causation to create anti causation. But using the body makes that fading away slower, that is a fact.

Let's Enlighten Specifications of The Types

The one we have been talking about; which has got many mitochondria and less nucleus which is changed to make aerobic (oxygenic) fermentation; and provide long term endurance is: Type I Muscle Fiber.

And the one; which has got many nucleuses, less mitochondria which is make anaerobic (non-oxygenic) fermentation; and provide short term excessive force strength is Type II Muscle Fiber.

But we mentioned Type IIa and Type IIb fibers. Type IIb actually is the one we are calling Type II all of this time. And Type IIa is a mix form between Type I and Type IIb.

Type IIa doesn't use ATP-CP energy source, it only uses glucose but in anaerobic form. In previous researches showed that;

Type IIb could be activated for 30-40 seconds at once depending on person.

Type IIa could be activated for approximately 6minutes at once.

Type I could be activated for many hours at once until you fade away or get tired which is a protective reflex of body.

As abstract, short explanation;

Person is using Type I; for walking and these kinds of soft actions. Also, people are using Type I muscles at most of inner organs activities.

Person is using; Type IIa for 3km marathon or casually running in the woods.

Person is using; Type IIb for 0 to 100 and 200 meters sprint runs or running away from a stray dog.

These fiber activations are like a 3 motored plane. To go on taxi way 1 motor might be enough. To go faster on taxi way, you have to start 2nd motor. And to fly off you have to start the 3rd and strongest one.

But as you noticed to start 3rd engine all of the engines have to be running already. And for to start 2nd engine you have to start first one before.

In muscles; First the Type I kinds are activated, if they cannot provide enough force 2nd ones are going inside to business. But if it is still not enough 3rd ones come after and all of them creates force at once. But obviously brain does understand this in less than a second and performs in less than a second. Thus, we never realize what's going on in muscles until the following day soreness. But what happens if all of these 3 muscle fibers are not enough to still take the flight get away. "The adaptation" occurs which will be explained in following topics.

Last Abstract of Physiology of Muscle

Number of fibers doesn't change, but ingredient of fiber changes, therefore fiber type changes. After fiber type change, the function and efficiency in occasions change as well. So, by changing causations which are workout or activity type those change fiber types; we are changing working purpose of human's body; which is essential to regulate on athletes, or anyone who want to do activities; or for the ones who wants to make their body perfect for long healthy life.

A powerlifter may get damaged by running for a long distance in low speeds. By damaging, it is meant; his achievement of lifting heavier. Because, the muscle will try to get smaller to spend less energy because of lengthen activity time causation, to make saving in energy. And for marathon runner it is not good to train with very heavy weights for short term. That makes muscles much less durable in energy consuming way.

There is no valid research on life expanding with the influence of muscle fibers. But there is one, to increase the life quality. Making activities and keeping muscles alive and functional making them last longer. Type IIb muscle existence is becoming a must in elders, because in elder phase of living; we are struggling with sitting, standing and climbing ladders. These kinds of activities are becoming Type IIb powerlifting activities due to decreased Type IIb sources and losing mass in every type of fibers with the age.

Squatting without weights are becoming a Type IIb activity in elders as well, because it requires 3 motors at once.

That is not about how much you lift, that is all about how much percentage of your muscle fibers required in the action. Evolution and revolution depend on that.

Energy Sources and Energy Usage of Body

Muscle Mechanism, Brain Functions and Muscle Types are introduced in previous topics. According to that information, every muscle fiber is different in a lot of ways from each other in the means of functioning. So that difference goes along with difference; in creation method, ingredients and energy usage method of theirs and along with them basal metabolism and brain functions.

At the beginning this has to be enlighten. Human body can use only 3 sources to create energy which are;

1- Fat
2- Glycose
3- Creatine Phosphate

There is always going on oxidative(aerobic) phosphorylation in body which occurs in the presence of oxygen in the cell and the process of breaking glycose to 36 ATP. When this ATP produce is not enough the 2nd and 3rd motors are getting involved such as in muscles and actually, along with muscle activity. Because, usage of all muscle fibers at once, requires peak amount of ATP in unit of time. Therefore, in order to create that much ATP, slow and long aerobic fermentation creation will not be enough. Body keep doing that but adding more sources aerobic phosphorylation(fermentation) in order to create more ATP, which is Anaerobic Fermentation and ATP-Creatine Phosphate Breakdown.

Anaerobic Fermentation and ATP-Creatine Phosphate Breakdown are not efficient way to use energy source due to creating 2ATP at one process of circle, but these are the ones which are faster and necessary in order to support, usage of ATP in unit of time.

In a table with usage priority;

1- Cellular respiration. Oxidative - Aerobic, Glucose to 36 ATP

2- Anaerobic Fermentation, converts glucose to 2 ATP

3- Creatine phosphate breakdown. anaerobic, recharges ADP to ATP.

Actually, body doesn't make a choose priority on these ones, but the actions make. If you force all of your muscle fibers at once, as %100 percent, then body goes up to all of 3 energy creating mechanism at once in less than a second.

As mentioned before, body is making first step of creating energy in base level for all the time which is **Cellular Respiration** due to base level of muscle fiber usage and internal organ usage. By adding 2nd level motors of muscle fibers to the action which are Type IIa or by increasing internal organ activity; specifically, brain activity body requires much more ATP in unit of time. Then, body must to start **Anaerobic Fermentation** along with cellular respiration. If, 3rd level motor activity which is Type IIb muscles are added to 1st and 2nd level motor muscle activation; body must start the 3rd energy creating source which is **Creatine Phosphate Breakdown** along with other two energy creating source metabolism.

1- Fat

Fat can be broken-down to ATP's. Fats cannot be converted into glycose in animal body which we have. Fat can only be digested, and ATP is yielded from them in 4 staged process. Which ends only with oxidative phosphorylation, which we mentioned as the longest but efficient way to use energy source.

Therefore, fat can't be used as a source of excessed body action but, can be used always in the base. Basal metabolism we call, which is using mostly fat molecules as its energy source. With every movement, walking, talking, sleeping we are using fat molecules. But increasing the basal metabolism and Type I motor activity we may increase the usage of fat molecules.

Fat only can be used in Type I motor activity and similar to that, most of internal organs' activity due to their long and 4 staged breaking process. But that doesn't mean Type I muscles and internal organs only can use fat molecules; they prefer it due to survival requirements of human body and genetic coding. But they may use glucose as well, when; there is increased glucose in the body or there is lack of fat molecules in the body.

Increased volume in activity or workout will not result with increased fat usage as it thought but it will result with increased glucose or ATP-creatine phosphate usage.

2- Glucose

It is the main source of anaerobic fermentation in the body. Human body is keeping glucose in the form of glycogen in the muscles and the liver. Body have got around of 400 grams of glycogen which may differ with gender, age, recent sports activity, weight. It keeps that in stores even a person has got 100 kg's of fat in its body. Because glucose usage is not optional it is essential with the increased volume of usage of muscles therefore involving 2nd level of muscle fibers into the action. Also, most of the brain activity requires too much ATP in unit of time like 2nd level muscle fibers do. That makes glucose essential for people who are using their brains more than the basal working rate, for that particular time.

2nd level of muscle fibers do not and cannot use fat as a main energy source due to needed high amount of energy usage in unit of time. They are already using fat molecules and it is not enough. Therefore, they make us of fat molecule and the glucose.

Glucose is the 2nd level of energy source and it is being added with the necessity of ATP even after usage of cellular respiratory capacity. Cellular respiratory is creating too much energy at once but when we degraded to in seconds base; it is not creating too much energy; it is the less form of creating energy when we degraded to unit of time base.

Glucose is mostly procured from carbohydrate. Actually, it is always procured from carbohydrate if there is no exceptional situation like starving to death. Overtaking carbohydrate, after filling all glycogen storages and blood flow of glycose; starting build of fat molecules in the body. Because glycose can be turned into fat molecules and it should, in order to continue to survivability of human. It is a long process, to be turned but there is no rush in that. Then, glucose can only be used as a source of fat by turning into that; like in the previous topic, in activity of Type I muscle fibers. Because there is no turning back, if it turned into fat; that almost always is being used as fat molecule in Type I activity and internal organs activity.

3- Creatine Phosphate

Creatine Phosphate is the main source of creatine phosphate breakdown which may be understood by its name. Creatine Phosphate storages are very limited in human body and they are not being used every day as energy source for non-sporting person. This breakdown is only activated in the necessary situations.

Creatine Phosphate Breakdown is the 3rd level of energy creating in the body and it only occurs in usage of the muscles in excessive volume which activates 3rd level of muscle fibers along with the other two.

Fat and Glucose metabolisms will not be enough to use more than %70 of muscle fibers. (percentage is different in every person, requires a biopsy to fully examine. In here it is given to understand the difference of 3rd level of muscle fibers.) Therefore, body is playing its last card which is Creatine Phosphate Breakdown.

ATP-CP breakdowns are not creating too much energy at total, but this process is the fastest of creating energy. Their biochemical structure is so weak that, this process takes a few seconds. Even total ATP creation is low with this process, when it is considered in unit of time creation of ATP, it is the most effective way to rapidly fulfilling the hunger of ATP. Therefore, they are needed to use in order to take the last step of the ladder.

Muscle Types and Their Energy Choice

Every muscle type stands for different kind of activation.

Basically, an abstract;

Type I for <u>hours</u> of working, slow but persistent work.

Type IIa for <u>minutes</u> of working, balanced between fast and persistent work.

Type IIb for <u>seconds</u> of working, fast but doesn't last a minute.

These function differences are based on their metabolic differences. As mentioned before; some of these cells have got many more mitochondria and some of them have got many more nucleus in their structures.

Therefore, their physiological working system and energy usage are different than each other.

Type I:

* Muscle is working as slow and for long term

* Rich of mitochondria

* **Slow and long process of creating energy**

* **Loves aerobic fermentation**

These last two bold phrases explain to the brain and to us. Why Type I should use FAT resource to create energy. Fat could be digested by mitochondria via its long and strong digestion. Known as Krebs cycle or citric acid cycle.

Due to this long digestion, none of the other muscle fibers could use fat as resource. Because those fibers need much energy in limited time due to fast twitching, high usage of energy in unit of time. Krebs (citric acid cycles) which is process of creating ATP from fat, could take many minutes.

During fresh start of long Krebs (Citric Acid Cycles); your Type I muscles could use some of ready-to-use ATP's in their cells. Because there is always aerobic fermentation, so Krebs, occurring in our body. With activation, number of fermentations are increased with the increased activity of Type I muscle fibers.

Body can't make the process faster, but body can increase the number of activated mitochondria, so number of fermentations at the same time. Therefore, when you start to aerobic exercise, many more of your mitochondria are being activated, and finally produced ATP's with oxidative fermentation are increased. That is why only oxidative(aerobic) fermentation lover Type I fibers can and should use Fat cells as an energy source while others not.

Type IIa:

* Muscle is working as fast and for mid term

* Rich of nucleuses and mitochondria

* **Fast and long process of creating energy**

* **Loves anaerobic fermentation**

These last two bold phrases explain to us; why this muscle should use Glycose as energy resource. So much energy required in limited time but for minutes. There is only one resource in body which can correspond this need, which is glycose. Because glycose's digestion is fast, this process happens in a few seconds. Also, glycose storages are much more than the ATP-CP storages in muscles and in body which will be explained in Type IIb. These storage in muscles could last longer 5-6 minutes. That is why, type IIa muscles last 5-6 minutes long in a single use. In resting time, muscle glycose storages are being refilled from glycogens. Glycogens are being teared apart to glycoses. It is a long process, but it starts with very first second of your exercises. Also, resting the body or limbs during these kinds of activities is not in seconds, it is in minutes. So that's why you have to rest in first place.

Type IIb;

* Muscle is working as fastest for short term

* Rich of nucleuses

* **Fastest and shortest process of creating energy**

* **Loves anaerobic fermentation**

These last two bold phrases explain to us; why this muscle should use Glycose and Creatine Phosphate as energy resource. Muscles is twitching very fast and needing energy in high amounts in very limited time for a short term. That kind of energy which is needed to be created in less than a second. Due to its biochemical structure ATP-CP can be broken-down in less than a second. There is no other energy source which can be digested in these limited seconds. Therefore ATP-CP is essential for Type IIb muscle. But this source is very limited in the cells. Therefore, it only lasts less than a minute. So, we have to rest the muscle to refill ATP-CP storages again. This resting process takes 2-3 minutes long optimally. But in sports, resting for 2 minutes not be the wisest move. But how much you get close to 5 minutes, that much storage refilled. It is a critic information.

All of these muscle fibers have got different sources of energy as it seems. But could they use other energy sources when they lack their main source?

The most critic knowledge on this topic is the answer of this question. And the answer is "No".

Their energy usage is accorded to the "time". They have to obtain energy within limited time of their muscle energy requirement, in per second or per twitch or etc.

Even though a person has got many kilograms of fat tissue, if there is not enough ATP-CP source in the muscle for that time, that person wouldn't be able to twitch his Type IIb muscles. That is why we cannot continue to twitch our muscles for unlimited time. Because their energy source drains after correct number of twitches, as it is mentioned. Particularly, whole source of Type IIb is drained maximally in 45 seconds of sprint running usage or you could think that as 6-8 repetitions in weightlifting activities. However, digesting one fat molecule takes more than minutes. This process wouldn't be able to support these muscles. And vice versa, even though ATP-CP storages or Glucose storages are filled, in usage of Type I muscle fibers they wouldn't be used. Because their energy creation is limited with being too fast in short time, but body needs long termed usage. If ATP-CP and Glucose were able to be used with Type I activity; marathon runners wouldn't be able to make a sprint at their last 100 meters after their whole marathon. Because they have been running for 2 hours and if they were had used their explosive power energy sources, they would be drained in a few minutes at the beginning of the race (Specially ATP-CP storages); and after the drain they couldn't run more than their regular 20km/per hour speed even in their sprints. But they are making their last sprints with 25-30km/per hour speed. So, that is a solid evidence of ATP-CP and Glucose storages in muscles are not being used during Type I activation no matter how long it is used.

As Abstract;

+ In Type IIb and Type IIa activity fat cells are not being used because lack of time to create energy.

+ In Type I activity glucose and ATP-CP storages are not being used because of not being preferred by brain, due to not being functional to the situation.

You could simply think that these 3 muscle fibers are 3 different type of Car Motors. *Gasoline, diesel and bioorganic.* A *gasoline* engine wouldn't work with *bioorganic* fuel and vice versa. These fibers are different type of motors and they use different fuels than each other. It doesn't matter how much gasoline you do have. This car doesn't burn gasoline because its motor is *bioorganic.*

Basically;

Muscle Fiber are in 3 Different levels and Energy Usages are in 3 Different Levels. Each Energy Usage Level stands for Each Muscle Fiber Level.

Muscle Type I = Cellular Respiration

Muscle Type I + Muscle Type IIa = Cellular Respiration + Anaerobic Fermentation

Muscle Type 1 + Muscle Type IIa + IIb = Cellular Respiration + Anaerobic F. + ATP-CP Breakdown

---

Note: Second and third equation written in cumulative form because of they are not being able to activate without %100 of previous muscle fiber type activation

Chapter 2:

General Health Systems In the Body

What is Fat?

Fat is a tissue. This part is very important, fat has not to be considered as a cell. Yes, there are fat cells in tissue, but fat is being stored as tissues beneath the skin and on the muscle. Fat doesn't integrate to muscles and placed between or around of muscles. It could be thought as three-layer system.

- First layer is muscle which is deepest when compared to other two.
- Second layer is fat tissue which could get very thick when forced.
- And third layer is skin which we can see from outside of the body.

Unused calories from fat and carbohydrate start to convert to fat tissue in a few hours but whole fat tissue process takes a few days.

However, there are some fat tissues which are placed around of internal organs such as heart and liver etc. Which usually overly-exist in unhealthy, over-weighted people. That internal organ fat has got levels. There is a common method to grade that level. On fat measure machines, which are working with bioimpedance measurements; as a result of machine; it is being showed. Which is starting from 0 to as it goes.

0 means there is no inner fat, and 13 is the maximal limit of internal fat. You may see higher numbers on that machine, but you shouldn't. That means it is going more than obesity.

If you go to the physician, you could hear that "you have got 2 grade liver fat formation." which is quite bad. Because on that scale which physician is talking, grading is going from 0 to 3.

Internal fat tissue generally related to a many kind of sicknesses or insulin resistance or whole-body fat level which is I will explain in our main caption.

In order to examine a person without any complicated measurements, you may look around of belly and how much he can hold with his hand when trying to take belly fat into palm. That is the additional fat which is a burden to body, and it shows the level of internal fat tissue; because of there is a relation between under skin fat tissue and internal fat tissue; due to genetic coded placement.

When Fat Tissue Increases and When It Decreases?

Fat increase in many occasions but, always there is one reason behind it. Unused calories. If you are taking much more calories than your body requires, that means your body going to store it. Because human body doesn't like wastage of supplies. Calorie is a supply which can easily be stored and used later. And calorie is the energy source of the body. Therefore, it is being used for 24 hour every day. It's not like proteins or other biologic supplies. Because your body not using all of the vitamins and minerals and proteins all day long. If human body is going to store these; vitamins, proteins and minerals there has to be a keen condition which is usually genetic code and workout.

As abstract; if you are taking much more calories than you spend in following time, those are going to be stored; in order to use later for same reason, when your body has got lack of calories. If you never go to lack of calories you will never use them.

As it is enlightened, this fat tissues decreases whenever there is lack of calorie from other sources in the blood and in your body. Because your body using calories in every single second. But sometimes this usage increases and decreases. Like in activity or in sports usage increases and while sleeping or watching television it decreases when compared to walking.

Partial Fat Losing

This is one of the most common desire. Losing fat as partial. Many people want to get rid of fat but only at particular places in their body.

But is it possible to lose fat as partial?

Every muscle is placed very far away from each other. When you think about your face muscles and leg muscles there is almost 1 meter between them. So, what about transfer between them? Even how far, these two muscles or two organs or two whatever are, there is always a way between them. Which is vein system. This system is so fast and so strong, it could always carry everything about human body in a few seconds. First of all, we have to keep in that mind to understand partial fat losing.

People could desire to lose their fat as partial. Probably many people would like to lose their belly area fat, and leg and arm fats etc. But it is not possible to lose them as only partial.

People are trying to work out or activate the muscles which are placed in the area that they want to lose fat. There are people in the gym who are all day and every day working out their abs, in order to lose belly fat. That is not how fat burning works.

Fat is not a tissue which bounded to muscle, fat is a tissue which bounded to body and veins. Fat is not integrated with muscles but as it mentioned, it is on the muscles and beneath the skin.

A person may think; for example, why an abs muscle cell would take the fat from arms, instead of nearest one to itself which is belly. Answer is so clear; your muscle never takes fat cell. Your liver takes them, digest them, turn them into pyruvate then release them to your blood system. Then your muscle takes the pyruvate and uses that in its mitochondria.

If body were going to take the nearest one in order to decrease the road time; body would take it from always around of belly. Because belly is the closest fat tissue to the liver.

Probably, the nearest fat tissue to the activated muscle; for many occasions such as face or arm activity, is the furthest one to the liver. Therefore, using those fat tissues which is furthest to the liver is the worst choice for the sake of system time.

"Does liver always use the nearest fat tissue to itself?". Of course not, body doesn't think things that simple. Human body is so complex and so intelligent than our consciousness. That is why we are still trying to figure out human body and developing sciences for that and not completely achieved yet.

While our body storing these fat tissues, it is considering many things. One of the major parameters is genetic code. Some people have most of their fat tissues in their cheeks or their buttocks or in their breasts. And some of them in their arms or belly. Everybody has got fat tissue almost in each body part yet, percentage of this storage's placement changes with genetic coding.

Second major parameter is your body always trying to keep your "center of mass" in same position which is; in males beneath the belly button when it is looked from forward, and to the symmetrical point when it is looked from the side. In female this point is placed a little lower.

Every kilogram placement in the body is so important to keep "center of mass" in the same place. Example; if somebody takes 3 kilogram of weight over its head near to back. He cannot; run, climb slopes or do many things. Because it is far away for body to protect the center of mass and "force effect" is calculated with "pathway x kilogram". That 3 kilograms weight in wrong place makes the same effect the 30 kilograms of weight in the right place in the terms of effecting the load on center of mass. Thus, your body tries to store many kilograms of these fat tissue near to "the mass center". Because it decreases the pathway therefore, the force effect to center. So that is why most of our fat tissue is placed around of buttocks, stomach, waist and upper legs.

The placement of fat around of body's center of mass, brings one huge benefit to people. Being able to live, function and survive with even 150 kilograms of fat tissue. People with mortal obese are even able to walk, climb stairs and so on. If their fat percentage was placed in their arms, legs or any other place which is far away to their center of mass, they wouldn't even able to move their limbs. With raising their arm, they would fall to that side, like a tumbler toy. Even if they don't fall, they wouldn't be able to move or use their limbs because of required excessive muscle power and endurance.

While losing fat or gaining fat we are always keeping the center of mass in similar area to being able to survive by moving and acting. That keep is made by same percental fat change in every limb and organ.

After these much explanation; That may finally be said: You cannot fight with your body's mind and your genetic codes. If you try manipulative ways to change that, your body always will compensate that to its origin.

Creation of human body is occurred according to too many parameters, and these are both two major ones. Fat losing is based on these explanations and that is why there is no partial fat losing in the body.

Fat Usage Mechanism

Your body uses the fat tissue in the same percentage when it placed over there. If a person has got 30 kilograms of body fat and %30 of these placed in belly area and %10 on face area and similar for other parts. Random person with these percentages; have got 9 kilograms of belly fat right now. When that person loses its 20 kilograms body fat with diet and only abs exercises, that person will still have his %30 fat in its belly area and %10 in face area. But the amount of fat mass around of belly will be decreased from 9kg to 3kg. He lost 20 kilograms at total but only lost 6 kilograms of belly area fat even though he is always doing abs exercises. He lost 14 kilograms from all of other areas with the percentage, which was the same in the first place and, decided by genetics and center of mass rule.

As mentioned before; muscles don't use fat directly and when person workout its abs, that doesn't mean the belly fat tissue will be digested first. It will be digested in same percentage with other fat tissues which are placed in all of the body.

Other Way Thinking

If a person still insists on the contrary idea after all of these explanations let's think in that way.

The theory:

"Body not using fat totally, but every muscle uses the nearest fat tissue or organ digest the nearest fat tissue to itself."

For this scenario: a person is always using its heart which works for 24 hours and 7 days. Then why still there is stored fat tissue around of its. Why not used that already? Also, heart fat tissue is one of the thickest ones in internal organs although it is the most working one.

In the muscle scenario, obese people have got huge cheeks in their face, even if they are salesperson and talking all day and every day. They are always using their face muscles, but they are keeping huge fat tissues in their face which we call as cheeks. But when they start to make diets and start to run, they start to lose their cheeks, along with the other body fat tissue in the body.

Correction and Final

"A person always stores fat tissue totally in the body and always uses fat tissue totally in the body. "

What is Blood?

Blood is the transfer vehicle of body which uses vessels as roads. If anything, goes through from one cell to another it has to be transferred via blood. Thus, circulation of blood effects everything in the body due to carrying everything about the cells.

Blood is carrying everything which is essential for the body. The energy sources, oxygen, hormones. Due to body's survivability is directly bounded to blood; the circulation has to be perfect in the body, otherwise all the systems in the body may be affected immediately.

This circulation is directly related with the condition of vessels and heart.

What is Heart?

Heart is the pump of the blood system. Circulation continues as long as it continues to work. There are 4 rooms in heart. Two of them are atriums and the other two are ventricles. Atriums; accept returning blood to the heart then transfer that to the ventricles. Then ventricles pump this blood to the body. The reason behind of this two-staged process is, heart has to regulate pumped blood amount at every turn. But heart cannot control incoming blood amount. So, it accepts and stores incoming blood in atrium then transfer the right amount to the ventricles.

Normally, in a normal person, ventricle pumps 80ml blood to body every second. Which makes approximately 5 litres of blood per minute. So, almost all of our blood cycles in our body are completed in a minute. This process is this fast; not because hormones have to circulate as this fast, but oxygen requirement has to be fulfilled constantly. Most of our cells use oxygen every minute so they have to meet with oxygen in their time. Also, energy sources have got hurry.

We never say that which step is the beginning step of this cycle but if we have to create steps in order to understand: First step; blood goes through capillary vessels of lungs, specifically alveolus, then take oxygen molecules via basic diffusion. Second step is coming to atriums and third is going to ventricles. Fourth is going and cycling whole body and fifth is coming back to heart in order to start to first step again. Big and small blood cycles are abstracted in this paragraph.

Changes in Heart

Heart goes through changes as physically (apart from emotionally) after some external events. Which might be happened in short or long term.

In Short Term, making a muscle or another cell usage more than its normal; that cell will require much more oxygen or glucose; therefore, will require much more blood to make interaction with. To bring much more resources to muscle; this cycle will get faster, because blood's carriage in per millilitre is limited. To make this cycle faster heartbeat rate will increase during the action phase.

If this kind of condition continues for many times and days, body will analyse this situation and will decide to make this process easier for heart muscle in the long term. Because, heart is being challenged and, body always must adapt to situation. Henceforth, heart will grow its ventricles limits, the storage and volume of ventricles. Thus, output of ventricles will increase for every pump. As a result, heart won't need to go over beat-rate of itself; because it will be able to complete the same blood cycle in a minute with lesser beating. Simply: *"100 times beating"* in a minute with 80 millilitres blood each time is equal to; *"80 times beating"* in a minute with 100 millilitres blood each time.

Heart muscle might get stronger and be able to push much more blood in once; stronger and better than we talked before as 80ml capacity. This amount is different for everybody depending on their lifestyle, activities and genetics. Heart will choose to get stronger in order to prevent going over the limit of beat-rate per minute.

Heart has got a maximum beating rate in a minute which is basically calculated as "220-Age". Heart never wants to go over this number. Because heart can't bear that burden. That burden we know as heart failure. Getting stronger and bigger of ventricles is the Long-Term change of the heart which is necessary to prevent heart failure with that kind of lifestyle, because body adapts to lifestyle, if right causations are given.

Heart Failure

Heart is an always working system from birth to death. That makes this system magnificent. But even this magnificent system has got its limits. Generally, there is an equation for this limit which is; 220-Age = Maximal Heart Rate. If heart reaches this rate and keeps going in this rate, that would make this system broken. Heart finally won't able to perform in that way or lesser way due to over-working and, it will stop. If a person keeps heart in safe limits this organ can work for a century or more. But pushing %100 of limit and trying to reach more than that for a significant time period, will break this system. Heart will try to beat many more times than %100 of limit itself for a minute or around that and its autonomous system will get into shock, not will be able to continue in healthy way, so will stop. And that is heart failure. That last minute generally happens on floor in pain. That case may final with not stopping and regulating itself as well. But it is completely uncontrollable.

Safe Beat Limits

Safe beat limit is %85 of maximal heart beating number, if that person not an athlete. In athletes %95 of that is acceptable while talking about safe limits. Obesity, cholesterol agglomeration, hypertension are the factors; which must be considered in order to lower "the %85 of maximal limit", so the safe limit. These numbers usually are reached in working out and high intensity activities.

Heart Development

Heart development could be commented as improving working limits of heart. Bearing much more blood output in a minute. It is necessary for a person which activates his body from time to time. Generally, athletes develop their hearts, with the exercises which known as cardiovascular exercises. Which is increasing output/per minute of heart also vessels' blood bearing power for per pump. These exercises have to be made by normal people to increase their heart health and durability. Both for athletes and sedentary people it has be done in an order. Because eventually heart is a muscle too and it has to be developed, as being controlled in the light of scientific information or trial-and-error information. The error that mentioned is; an incident which result with death or not achieving development of heart, which figured out in the past, before sophisticated science elements.

With the light of sophisticated science researches, we can clearly say that; This heart development; in sedentary person can be made at %70-85 and for athletes at %80-95 of maximal beat rate levels of heart as optimally. A person has to keep heart rate stabilized in these ranges to induce to development in heart. This stabilization process has to be in minutes preferably more than 15 minutes. Also, not only for once, it has to be done for days and months consecutively. Because, as it has been said, it is a long-time and consecutive process to make an adaptation of improvement in the whole body or a part of the body.

As abstract; likewise, everything else in body. You have to use one element of the body by pushing its limits for long-term to get an improvement. It is same in all of muscles, all of organs, even for brain the same rule applies.

Decreasing in Heartbeat Rate

Heart Volume will decrease during resting compared to before, after its development occurred. For example; a normal adult resting Heart Rate per minute is around of 60. But if this person is an athlete who developed its heart, the resting Heart Rate per minute might be around of 40. Because in "development", ventricle growth is occurred permanently (With the condition that; person continues to same kind of activity and keeps same causation in the field). After this growth, blood volume with per pump is increased. With this increase if heart continues to pump blood to body with same beating rate, the circulation of blood will be unnecessarily high for the requirement of the body and body is not after waste of energy to make unnecessary heart beats. Therefore, heart finds the solution by decreasing Heartbeat Rate/Per Minute. And keeps total circulation of blood volume at the required level with lesser beatings.

Benefits of Growing Ventricles and Vessels

Due to increased blood volume at per pump; body will able to pump more blood with lesser heartbeat. Therefore, in activity heart rate will drop to lower numbers as well as the in resting heart rate does. Thus, reaching the maximal heart rate will be much harder for body. In other saying, body's activity level is increased or is being less limited or not limited with blood reaching capacity to the tissues.

We may increase the per pump volume, but we are not able to increase maximal heartbeat capacity which is related with genetics and age. That is why ventricles' volume and vessels' volume improvements have to be acquired in order to increase cardiovascular (Heart&Vessel) capacity, henceforth the body's maximal exercise and activity capacity.

Exercise and activity capacity are bounded to many parameters, but cardiovascular capacity is one of the most critical ones. If it is not good related with other parameters, it is making a bottleneck effect and limits whole capacity.

Heart Growing

"Heart growing is bad!" it's a common sense. But it is a minus sentence. Because as it is explained; heart needs to grow to increase clean blood output per pump. By saying growing we are referring to atriums and ventricles. But growing in heart is bad when it happens in septum. Which means walls of the heart. Generally, in people "Septum Interventricular" grows as a disease. Growing of septum might be expected because of growing of ventricles. But in this heart disease; septum which placed between ventricles, called as septum interventricular, grows excessively. And that makes hearts movement harder also this growing makes ventricle capacity smaller. Because the Heart doesn't grow from outside, but it grows tissue from inside. That means the cavity inside of its will be smaller after this process occurs. That will make ventricles smaller therefore, heart will have to beat many more times per minute. Which were bringing us "The Heart Failure" during the activity.

As Abstract; Heart growth is good if occurs with presence of sportive activity, but excessive septum growing is bad in whichever condition.

Blood Pressure

Blood doesn't have its own pressure in any way, because it's in liquid form. By saying blood pressure, the pressure of cardiac output is being referred. Ventricles pushing the blood so hard, it's almost like a garden hose inside of there and all of that pressure is being carried by veins. How much closer to the ventricle that much pressure occurs on veins. So, the biggest vein by capacity and thickness is "aorta". Because this one meets maximum amount of blood with maximum amount of pressure. And it has to be durable in order to not ripped apart with effect of pressure. Because it is lifelong thing and that pressure increases and decreases from time to time. With pressure, a tension occurs on walls of veins. If this tension goes too high, it is being called "hypertension" and if it goes too low it is called as "hypotension". Both of are a kind of sicknesses if they are occurring frequently.

Human's heart output pressure decreases or increases. We cannot measure that pressure. We can measure the pressure in our veins. And we say, "Your tension is high or low.". By saying this, we are talking about tension in veins which attribute to cardiac output.

There is a limit of this tension/pressure bearing by veins. Generally, it is known as; 120mm/80mm mercury is ideal in our home tension measuring devices which is sphygmomanometer. When pressure goes to high, vessel's walls get flexible. 220mg mercury of systole (the bigger number) is the maximal limit which vessel walls can get. If you go near or over of this limit, walls cannot bear that much tension and be damaged. In long term that damages become a tear in veins which is lethal. Reaching this much is not necessary, a bit of high for long term may damage the walls as well.

The tension decreases in external veins due to being far away to source of output. But symptoms still could be seen in external veins. Generally, in kidneys' and brain vessels. People might feel a pain on these areas according to hypertension on its veins. But not always it has to be felt. Sometimes a human can tear a vein apart without noticing. And realizes that, after seeing internal bleeding symptoms. Commonly, nose bleeding a good example. Those veins are too weak and with even a bit of hypertension may affect them.

Hypertension might be cured with ease if it is not occurred in a rare way such as mutation in embryo form. Even in that kind of occurring, it can be cured with some manipulators which can enlarge vessel roads by enlarging its walls as temporarily, which are medicines.

Hypertension might be cured as permanently in an organic way which is using and improving the heart and vessels which we know as cardiovascular system. We are always using them but, they needed to be challenged in safe limits which is mentioned as till %95 or %85 limits or lesser in special conditions. It is easy to measure %85 limit of the heart because of; the devices that shows heart rate and, we are already knowing the maximal rate. In the veins side, we cannot calculate simultaneously the extension of veins and we don't even know its maximum limits. But we may see some symptoms such as redness on eyes, pain in the kidney's, heart or head and usually headache which continues for a while. These symptoms usually are the caller of hypertension in vessels and due to overextending in walls; occurred pain which felt.

Challenging will improve vessels' effectivity by making them larger as permanently in long-term. Challenge with activity in safe limits, which we may call as workout. Cardiac workout may be done with any kind of exercises which increases heartbeat and tension. Because without a significant increase in these two; body will not be challenged therefore, will not adapt itself to the new situation which is wanted.

Hypotension is a sickness as well, was mentioned before. In hypotension blood cannot go through veins efficiently and blood circulation get slow. That makes people dizzy and fading away. Sometimes after sitting for a long time or after waking up, when you stand up your sight starts to become black, and you become dizzy. That is because your tension is decreased due to inactivity for a long time and cannot reach the blood to tissues effectively. Due to lack of sources which comes via blood, body starts to lose some functions which brings as dizziness kind of symptoms. Hypotension is usually treated manipulation of medicines or manipulation of food; it usually requires continues treatment of such kind. Because hypotension never occurs with overactivity or that kind of thing, body would always create a balance between heart performance and total tissue mass in the body. Hypotension is usually related with known or unknown sickness factors.

Oxygen Saturation

O_2 Saturation is basically; the percentage of haemoglobin with oxygen compared to all haemoglobins. This number can be measured from finger. Many basic devices have got this feature.

Normally the saturation has to be between %90 and %100. If it is going lower than these numbers, there may be a problem about capillary system of lungs or breathing or heart. It effects every kind of performance of the body due to everything in body works with oxygen, bounded to that with blood.

What is Flexibility?

Flexible is a word for, being able to; lengthen then being able to shorten. Human body is flexible in the most ways but as limited. It is limited because of the structure of its components.

Human body contains many structural components, such as; bones, muscles, ligaments, tendons, joint capsules etc. However, not all of them are flexible such as bones and tendons. Also, some of them flexible but in a very limited amount, such as joint capsules. And some of them are the main element of being flexible such as muscles.

Neutral Form of Muscles

With every movement, muscles are shortened and lengthened. While standing still in comforted position, that's the neutral position almost of every muscle which is, muscles are neither shorten nor lengthen, therefore not creating any force. In this form they don't get any damage which is related with activity or they don't use energy more than necessary amount and enough to continue their base contraction and living expenses.

Every movement creates changes in muscles or as

correct saying; every change in muscles creating movements. This movement may be in the way of result of muscle contraction or it may occur in the opposite way of subject muscle. If it is being in the way of muscle contraction it is called as flexing and if it is being at the opposite way to muscle contraction it is being extending. Actually, the term of "flexibility" is used for the limit of that extension. How much extension capacity muscles have got, that much the body is able to see challenged angle limits in its joints; therefore, much extreme movements.

Flexibility: Adaptation in Long Term

Being shortened and lengthened have to be in limits. The bands between muscle fibres deciding amount of how much muscle will be flexed or extended in total. Ability to shorten and lengthen much more can be improved in time with workout.

As we know many rhythmic gymnastics athletes have got too much lengthen limit due to improving their in-muscle bands' lengthening limits; therefore, its muscle flexibility. However, strength trainers such as bodybuilders are improving their muscle shortening ability with their exercises without purpose.

Both of shortening and lengthening has got limits and both of these limits may be increased. Flexibility trainings are being made with lengthening so extending muscles. Which is commonly known by everyone but will be explained as detailed in this section.

Shortening trainings which are known as strength trainings will be explained in other sections, but one critical thing about it; making shorten and challenging muscle in shortening way increases its shortening capacity therefore the force it can produce with the movement.

After mentioning long term flexibility, mentioning about short term flexes has to be done.

Flexing: Short Term

With every movement we are flexing and extending few muscles as it is mentioned. But these flexes and extends have acute effects on the cells. These effects' types change according to the form of the movement type.

Flexibility is an ability of a muscle which is earned in long term with extending it. How to extend muscle to gain flexibility? Which kind of flexibility or are we gaining opposite of flexibility?

A movement which is; Fast or slow, for long or short period, by pushing maximum or not are the factors that make different between flexibility types. Following three titles are showing types of flexibility gaining methods and what kind of flexibility that is giving.

A) Static Extending; Known as Static Stretch

Extending muscle fibers;

As Slowly

For Long Period

By Pushing limits to the maximum but gradually.

This extend is being used, to take two outcomes.

a) To lengthen the muscle fiber in the long term by repeating it. As gymnastic athletes do.
b) To help regeneration after any kind of workout. This stretch helps to moving metabolic wastes such as carbon dioxide and lactic acid. Using this method immediately after workout of the muscle helps the regeneration as major and increases the performance of the muscle in following day.

Specific note for this stretch: It has to be done equal and more than 30 seconds in every turn. Less than 30 seconds doesn't give these effects according to most of the authorities.

To lengthen muscle fiber permanently: this process may go until minutes. While performing stretches, to reach the maximum limit and a bit more than that; help of another person or machine may be used; this method is usually applied by gymnasts.

B) Ballistic (Active) Extending: Known as Dynamic Stretch

Flexing and Extending muscle fibres;

As Fastly

For Short Period

By Pushing limits to the maximum and more at once.

In this stretch we are making flexion with opposite (agonist) muscles of subject muscles. With the fast flexion of the opposite muscles, subject of stretch muscle's fibers are being extended with a force for short time. Trying to kick the roof, like soccer players do is one of good examples to this stretch. They are activating their hip flexor muscles hereby; they are extending their hip extensor muscles with an excessive force at the end of the movement.

This form of stretching is being used for three metabolic and functional improvements.

a) To increase metabolism of the muscle. By making these stretches, extended muscle fibres are being used very effectively and that creates a necessity of oxygen and energy source in muscles. That necessity fastens the heart and vascular system activity and also metabolic activity of related muscle fibres. Improving the metabolism in this way, prepares the body and muscles for further activities in following minutes.

b) To increase contractibility of the muscles. Because contracting them as fast in maximum limits, creates a big force on them which activates most of the muscle fibres. Therefore, nervous system from brain to muscles and neuromuscular junction are being activated. And muscles are being prepared to contract against forces or with conscious contracts of muscle which will be performed in following minutes.

c) To Increase opposite muscle's preparation for further ballistic movements. Because muscles are being injured during activities because of; the movements those occur which body is not used to it, or with the movements which are too extreme for muscles. By making this kind of extreme stretches to the muscles; activate muscle's brake system which is eccentric contraction. The contraction in the opposite way to the movement in order to slow and stabilize movement.

These three activations are beneficial for athletes or any kind of sportsman in order to warm up to the exercises and also prevent muscle injuries which are occurring due to muscle and tendon unawareness.

C) Functional Flexibility: Known as Functional Stretch

Flexing and Extending muscle fibres;

as Fastly

For Short Period

By Pushing limits to the maximum and more.

Extension of muscles in this method same with dynamic stretching. But the difference between two of them is; in functional flexibility, movements are formed according to the following movements. This stretching is being in the similar pattern with the upcoming activity. The reason of this and difference between dynamic is;

a) To improve and prepare neuromuscular system for upcoming activity.

This stretch has to be performed with lower stress than the actual movement. Otherwise it would be the movement' itself. And lowering the stress has to be with the way of lowering weights that is going to be lifted or the forces on body which are placed in order to increase stress and challenge it. If fiber extension or flexion speed or period is different; that wouldn't be beneficial for the upcoming movement. So, the stretch has to be in the exact same form of the movement.

What is Posture?

Posture is basically can be explained as bodies' and limbs' stance against gravity with neutral standing position of every joint while standing still on feet.

Skeletal system is not able to stand by on its own. If we put a human skeleton on its feet, it would immediately drop to the floor. The thing that is giving them human posture is muscular system.

Muscles pull the bones from the points where they attached. This pull is happening according to muscle's linear positioning. Muscle always pulling bones to the specific position which is the other attachment point of muscle which is to another bone or tendon. So, muscles keeping two bones together and tight to each other. But there is also, another muscle is attached to the same bone from another point of attachment and other end of the second muscle is attached to another bone which apart from the one we have talked about. That muscle is pulling the main subject bone to the other end of its. There is a sweet fight between these muscles if they are attached in the opposite ways.

There may be more than 3 attached muscles on a bone and makes it more complex to understand. All of them pulling the bone in different directions, with contraction few of these muscles' and with the occurred movement. If every attached muscle are contracted at the same time, if they are in the same strength or contracted in same strength there will not be any movement in the bone therefore in the limb or the body as we see from outside.

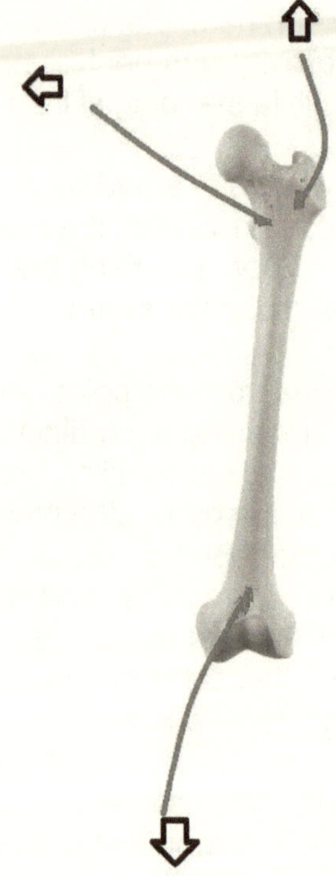

This picture is not exactly related with any muscle or bone in human body. It is only put due to demonstrate how bone may be pulled in many directions, or a few directions at the same time.

Not a single bone makes a difference in body if it is not a big specific one like humerus or femur which is the only bone of upper arm and upper leg. But even for those big ones, there are many things has to be considered about their posture. The posture of bone may be about its own related muscles or not. If it is its own muscles, it is easier; to understand the posture, the changes those has been occurred in posture and correcting the posture. But if it is related with other related bones or muscles, it makes the situation much more complex.

How to Observe Posture?

While observing postural changes or if posture is correct, all of the possibilities always should be considered. From toe to head every joint has to be examined. Because all of the skeletal system is a chain which has got not break point. From toe to head every bone is attached with each other with joints and they are standing with the factor of muscle tissues. The change which occurred in the feet even may affect the spine's bended posture which is known as scoliosis.

Every bone and muscle in the body are related with core area which is close to belly button. It can be considered as symmetry point of weight and strength, that is actually why we call it core muscles. Every joint and limb has to be observed, then the other attached to that one has to be observed; step by step until reaching the core. This observation may also start from core to be examined through the last bone of the limb or to the bone which is changed in the terms of posture.

There are always two sides in the body. Front and back or right and left or top and bottom. All three; "bottom and top "or "right and left" or "front and back" sides have to be close to core area as equal both in terms of strength and weight. Even if it is not made with consciousness, it is being done by brain with time. If you get much more belly fat your core point, mass center will move to the front for a bit, in order to balance center of mass and bring that back to its original position; body takes your upper back to much behind. People don't realize it until someone says, "Your belly comes to the room then you come." It is not only related with big belly, but their head and upper back are standing at much more behind than usual. This one is an occurred postural change along with the center of mass of the body; it didn't happen in one day and we are not doing it with consciousness. It is a process. A process of changing in muscle posture therefore body posture.

What is Tonus?

Tonus is the contraction of the muscles which keep them hard and active which is necessary to have a body form. Without tonus we can't keep any posture. Dead people losing their tonus, and that's why it is so hard to carry them without a cabinet, they are becoming a loose weight. With the age, tonus of muscles is decreasing. People are becoming less durable to external effects, having difficulty to give reflects, and losing their balance easily in elder ages.

Tonus is the main factor why skeletal system has got shape even while sleeping or walking. Because every muscle is contracted for some, which is enough to keep body in a customized form and carry it.

All of the muscles are always contracted at some percentage even if we don't use them actively, Different percentage of contraction is equal to different muscle length. Muscles have bands in them which are crossly shaped. These bands are getting into each other with every contraction and getting shorter. Even they are not contracted they are into each other for some. And the amount of being into each other while resting with only power of tonus decides the resting length of the muscle. Shortened or lengthened muscle length is equal to more approximated or separated bones which we call as change in the posture.

The tonus, the muscle's base contraction may be different for everybody. It may differ according to the age, activity and exercises level, gender, genetics. Even for same person, this percentage is different in every muscle. While sleeping or standing still, a person's abs muscle may be contracted with %17 of all muscle fibers' power while lower back muscles are %14 contracted. Which is a reason of muscle imbalance and therefore with changed bone relation and body shape; the postural problems. The critical action to take in order to fix this is, either growing muscles of the weak side or increase the contractibility of week side and decrease the contractibility of strong side which we know as changing the tonus.

What Changes the Posture and Muscle Posture?

1) Muscle mass increasement changes posture, no matter how much they want to be in low tonus at every fiber; in total, complete muscle tonus will be much stronger for posture than before. Because 10 millimeters of fibers with %10 tonus is better than 5 millimeters of fibers with %15 tonus. By the millimeters of fibers; we are referring muscle fiber mass, the cross-section.

2) Working out muscles increases their tonus, due to adaptation for being ready to workout anytime. Because body thinks it is a commonly used muscle. And it always has to be stronger and faster.

3) Overusing the muscles, changes the position and form of the joints. Also, overusing one muscle increases its tonus as well. Increased one muscle's tonus without increase in opposite of that leads to change in bone's position.

4) Keeping same posture for a long time is a form of overusing. The office workers usually have got humpback, which is because they always keep that humpback posture and that creates a new posture on them. Because we may be born with some genetics, but they may externally change with force of the time. The time which passed in same conditions for too long. These conditions actually are; the changed tonus of the muscle, by making some muscles shorten we are increasing their tonus permanently, therefore the long-term posture. The excessive shortening of muscle for once is equal to movement in human body. We are always shortening at least a muscle while we are moving a limb while we are also lengthening the opposite muscle of that.

5) Genetics is a recently found factor of wrong posture. People who have got scoliosis or spine change related hernia, also have relatives in the same conditions. Specially, a teen girl has got scoliosis, her sister usually having it due to scoliosis is being transferred in "X" gene.

6) Bone mutations, such as impingement of acromion bone. Bones are getting in a form by mutations which they shouldn't be. The reason of this is still grey for science but we know one thing: these changes bring some different development in the limbs and joints. Muscles comply with the situation and posture changes.

Static and Dynamic Posture

Posture had been explained as bodies' and limbs' stance against gravity with neutral position of every joint while standing still on feet. But we are not always standing still on feet.

Human usually in a movement either it is major or minor. During this movements our limbs so our joints are moving. Their relationship with body, their standing to the core is changing. This posture is important as much as standing still one.

Dynamism should be performed in safe human body dynamism limits. Safe meaning; which is not bringing any deficiency to the body with excessive repetition. It should be remembered; these limits may be improved with workout in time. If it is not performed in the limits this may can defined as "Wrong Dynamic Posture".

Wrong dynamic posture may occur due to wrong consciousness of person. Such as trying to lift a very heavy object from the floor without bending the knees but only bending the lumbar spine. That kind of lifting increases the load in the lumbar spine due to a basic physics rule. Further to the lifting center equal to heavier load. Weight is being multiplied with road to the load. The lifting center is lumbar spine in this kind of lifting and that much of created load event with light weight due to wrong posture, will change its components in undesired way.

Wrong dynamic posture also may occur because of wrongly learned movement patterns by brain. One of the common one is bending body forward while making squats. Body is making this compensation in order to protect center of mass in front. By making this, body is loading the weight to the upper leg muscles which are trusted mainly by brain. Because those are very strong muscles in everybody due to commonly daily usage by everyone. This compensation is being apart from consciousness. This kind of wrong movement patterns may create a deformation with many repetitions in time.

Changed dynamic posture may not always be considered as wrong. Specially for sportsmen or special conditioned people, it may be necessary. It will be explained as detailed in the following titles.

What Happens If Posture Changes?

Static posture is important because we are keeping that form for most of the time, and static posture is explained as on the feet posture but; sitting still or driving a car or these kinds of action are static posture as well. They just do not be placed in the definition in order to not make that more complicated. Humans spend most of their times in static posture and with the impactful effect of the time, static posture may be deforming for joints, tendons, muscles or even bones.

Joint positions and movement of joints will change. Over time some joints may not get along with that in healthy condition. Common example; shoulder. If you strengthen your chest muscles way more than upper back muscles, it would take your shoulders to the forward because of increased muscle tonus. With the time, keeping glenohumeral(shoulder) joint in forward will squeeze some departments in joint gaps because lack of space to fit. It may occur during the movement or even without movement depending on the level. Finally, it will bring some kind of injuries which is hard to fix because main reason; the posture has to be fixed first and it takes time.

Lifting heavy objects in wrong form in the terms of bending and performing squats with bended back, may create a hernia in the lumbar disks even if a person has got perfect form in its static posture. Because during the time person is making actions, load is being added to that particular joint because of changed form. That is increasing the impact on joint. Even without external weight addition or wrongly formed joints; because of changed load road, body itself may be an additional weight for some joints. Every joint has got its limits to bear in correct form of usage and in incorrect form of usage. Usually that bear amount is very lesser in incorrect form lesser than correct one. Due to changed posture during dynamism, load is being borne in incorrect form. Therefore, deformation occurs.

Game has to be played according to its rules. Body and physic have got its limits and rules, so we have to play along with them. It is the only way to not get into a deformation or pain which occurred because of biomechanical reasons such as posture changes.

How to correct posture?

By rebalancing agonist (directly related with subject muscle) and antagonist (contra activist muscle of the movement or muscle) muscle balances. As in shoulder agonist muscles of forward shoulder is pectoralis major and minor which we know as chest muscles. Antagonists of them are rotator cuff and rear deltoid muscles. So, rebalancing total tonus of them will fix the issue. It is same in every joint of body. Rebalancing the tonus of the muscles in desired way is the only organic treatment of wrong posture if it is not related with bone mutations. Even if it is related with bone mutations rebalancing the muscle biomechanism would solve the situation in general.

There are some special issues. We call them special but actually they are quite common. Increasing the tonus of rear deltoid and rotator cuff not might be enough because it will close distance between shoulder blade with glenohumeral joint (Shoulder Joint). But not will close the distance between shoulder blade and spine. If that distance is wide, closing others won't be enough, shoulder will still be in front. That distance has to be approximated as well. So, as it mentioned before; examination has to start from; the joint, which is not standing correct, through the core area. Everything between of them has to be evaluated.

Closing distances and approximating bones or separating distances and abducting bones may be done in two ways;

a) Increasing or decreasing the muscle mass or effectivity of specific muscles. Which may be done with concentric exercises. By shortening muscle with presence of load on that and therefore increasing its limits as physiologically in time. Weight workout is perfect example for it. To decrease the gap, leaving muscles passive and not making activity or exercises with them is the organic way of decreasing the muscle mass, therefore the total cumulative tonus.

b) By increasing the specific muscles' tonus which is wanted to be shortened or decreasing the specific muscles' tonus which is wanted to be lengthened.

How to Change the Tonus?

It is mentioned that tonus of few muscles has to be "strengthen" or few of them has to be "weakened" or both of them at the same time in order to change posture. This weakening and strengthening is happening for the base level of the muscle contraction, it is not the top level, maximal contraction; we wouldn't want to change that. That stands for maximal power and strength.

a) Increasing

Strengthening the base level of contraction or in other saying, increasing the tonus may be done by isometric contraction of muscles. It is a term in order to classify contraction type of muscle.

Isometric name is coming from isolating the metric attribute. So, anything may change in the muscle, except its metric attribute; which is length. There are two types of contraction. Isometric is the directly related one with tonus increasement.

Contracting the muscle without changing the muscle length; therefore, not actually doing any movement under load; is when this type of contraction occurs. It may still be seen from outside that muscle is getting harder and getting tired to keep that form under load. Carrying a fruit case is a perfect example for this one. Arms are only holding it still without doing any movement but they still getting hard and tired after a while.

Isometric contraction activities may be done in daily life, also they may be adapted to exercises as well.

Dynamic type and functional type of stretching will increase the tonus, due to their powerful contraction creation during and in end phase of the movement. They may be applied as tonus increasement exercises.

However, there is no necessity to choose only one of the increasement methods. Both isometric exercises and concentric exercises may be performed at the same protocol of changing the posture; and it would give better results than performing only one at once.

b) Decreasing

Decreasing muscle tonus may be done by stretching again, but only static stretching.

Static stretching for a significant time is stimulating Golgi tendon organs in the muscle. They are giving the stimulation; that the muscle is being challenged by its length and it has to get longer. Otherwise, muscle may get damage and muscle trying to adapt situation. Performing this repetitively will create permanent effect in muscle because of body's adaptation rule.

Significant time of static stretching to muscle is found as more than 30 seconds. Less than 30 second of static stretching at once is giving very lesser results compared to more than 30 seconds. But going over than 60 seconds is not changing the results significantly.

Is Wrong Posture Must Always Be Fixed?

All of the components of the body get used to posture after a while, either it is correct or not. Therefore, changing one of limb's posture may not be enough to correct whole posture. Also, due to spending too much time in wrong posture, other joints of the body which are related with wrong one, location of those may be changed or protocols of those may be changed due to be in accord with the wrong one. So, changing the wrong one, requires a new adaptation for the related ones, which may never occur. Most of the people who wants to change their posture; are living with that for many years, may be even from birth. This change may be seemed like a fixing, but other limbs and joints may not get along with that and that fixing may bring other problems with itself. Therefore, in these conditions not to fix posture may be considered.

Sportsmen who are; living for their profession and also successful in their job. They usually have got postural changes in their body depending on their sport. Flat foot in marathon runner is like a must, for many of the football players as well. It may increase their performance in their sports, because they are making something which is not human body designed for in the first place. Fixing these changes may decrease the effectivity of their body in their sport. Posture fixing may not be chosen in these kinds of conditions.

Pain or functional deficiency are the absolute determination factors. If there is pain in person due to changed posture such as flat lower back which brings hernia with itself, that posture should be fixed. Someone who can't elevate and turn his arm because of; humpback with narrowed shoulder gap along with pain of squeezed compartments in there. This one must be fixed too.

Yes, there is a perfect posture which may be draw in paper. But trying to bring everybody to that posture may not always be the best idea.

Improving Body Mechanism

Improving the functions of the body and thus potential of body mechanism is mainly about muscle usage. Because all of the movement is directly related with muscle and muscle is what makes human, different than a plant as mechanically. Muscle has to be worked proper according to the aimed movement; and neuromuscular system has to work in efficient way along with muscle.

Both of these can be improved in perfect way by exercises or making activities in correct order. This order may be thought as, upgrowing a baby. A baby learns to move its limbs then to stabilize them by using force; for example, standing on its arms then learns to move them against a force which is gravity or resistance of objects, then by getting stronger then make strength activity which is being able to throw objects or take itself on foot.

Proper form of improving the body mechanism is similar to improving steps of baby. As abstract, we are;

1- Improving our mobility, range of motions
2- Improving our stability, moving objects or ourselves in a stabilized way
3- Improving our strength, being able to move the heavier
4- Improving our power, being able to move as faster or quicker.

While evaluating and improving functionality of human body; the following headline must be considered.

Steps of perfect functionality;

It is similar to construct a building. If you make one floor weaker than it should be, the building will collapse eventually, without being bounded to whichever floor it is. So, body improvement has to be considered 5 staged process; but not everybody starts from the first stage and not everybody should have reach to last stage.

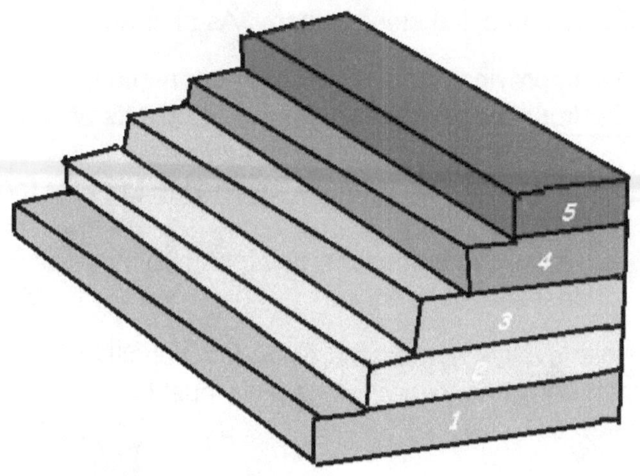

5 Floor Representing

1- **Mobility**
2- **Stability**
3- **Strength**
4- **Hypertrophy**
5- **Power**

It is a 5-floor representing because everything in body mechanism is being built on each other in this order.

Some of them may not be directly bounded to the one before, but in movement and functional status they are bounded to each other and the lower floor has to be improved first or along.

1. Mobility

Human mobility is limited. Mobility is a term used for "joint mobilities". Every joint has got its limits depending on genetics; even it is so good as genetically, it still has got a maximum limit. On the other side, minimum mobility of a joint could be zero. It might be a joint something like in cranium (skull) which disappear after infancy and become bone's itself; or it could be a lifelong joint like shoulder which may lost its mobility due to deformities in joint with some traumas or long-time immobility or diseases such as rheumatoid arthritis and may become immobile.

Joint has got its maximum limit without tearing apart its capsules or damaging itself. There is one more limitation factor on mobility apart from deformities; which is normal shape of the joint and bones and injuries, affected directly by muscle tension. Joint mobility is based on muscle tension which muscles are related with that particular joint. Increasing muscle tension (tonus) will limit the maximum flexibility range of muscle and it will result as less mobile joint.

There are two factors on increasing joint mobility which can be considered as two steps. First step is joint's health. Even though a person's muscles are most flexible muscles in the human history if there is any issue in the joints such as rheumatoid arthritis;

motion will be limited by that. Else, joint capsule may not be that much dynamic; it has to be gained some dynamism first. Then, the second factor should be considered which is muscle tension.

Due to being immobile for long time, genetic factors or working out the muscle in shortening way, result of shortened muscle is taken which is another definition for tensioned muscle. Tensioned muscles are not allowing bones to not move in long range; thus, we call related joint as less mobile joint.

To increase Mobility both factors have to be increased.

- First step is, health problems in the joint; decreasing inflammation in joint, increasing dynamism of joint with rehabilitation techniques or flexibility training have to be done.

- Second step is, decreasing the tension of muscle. Which can be done with some pharmacological help or with a surgery technique which called rhizotomy (generally done in diseases related with un proper using of nerves) and finally the most natural way and preferred method; stretching in correct form and time. Stretching is giving its effects in long term, but it is completely natural and harmless. This method is explained in flexibility and posture titles as detailed.

2. Stability

Stability of human is essential as much as mobility in order to live a life with quality. Stability might be considered as "Whole body's stability" or "Individually for every joint". To; make a standing stance, pick, push, pull and every other action requires related joints' stability in some way. Every living multijointed organism develop its stability skills from born. But it is a lifelong skill which developed for every joint individually. It has levels, depending on person and joint.

Stability of joints are related to muscles which embracing it. There is always a force on the joint in every action. This action may be pulling, pushing, rotating or everything. Direction of force always changes, perpendicular, horizontal, diagonal or mix of everything. Human perception system is not fast and capable enough to analyze and create an answer on these forces, but nerve system is. Human body always goes into shock when it meets with a force for the first time. Then it starts to learn that kind of force and how to react. Every repetition makes it better and smoother.

Reaction to the force becomes smoother because; frequency of nerve stimulation is increased due to create more fitting answer. Nerve system creates a memory special for that force and for that muscle. Because with even a few repetitions it wants to adapt for further repetitions which is expected naturally due to survivalist capacity of body and adaptation philosophy.

How much it learns the movement and the force that much response stimulations it can create. Therefore, can keep the joint in the position that is wanted to be. Because force is not a singular thing comes once and goes away. Even the force is applied less than one second, it is a process; and answer of body to that actually is summation of all the forces and responses.

Experiencing the muscle – nerve usage for repetitions in a muscle is may called as educating the muscle.

In educated muscle, educated in the terms of being able to efficiently use it, there are hundreds of analyses and contractions occurring in a few seconds. We see all of those in a one smooth movement. If amount of contractions decreases due to not being used with the movement or another physiological reasons, we start to see a shaking during movement. Decreased frequency in contractions also decreases the smoothness of movement. If muscle trying to prevent the movement with those hundreds of contractions in less than a second, we see a perfect stability in the joint no matter what is the effect. If it is not making contractions with enough frequency and power, we start to see a shake of the joint with the effect of force.

Better stability is protecting joint against big shakes which can lead to injuries during big traumas such as landing from a high jump. Even there is no big force as in jumping, better stability always provides better weight disruption in the joints, therefore it provides the protection of components of the joint, against wrong and continues usage of the joint and its components. Thus, it prevents cumulative injuries such as some forms of arthritis.

Stability is important for every sportsman in order to not get injured or create better force. Getting injured happens mostly because of excessive movement in joint or in muscle which is not expected. Being able to keep these in the safe range and form would always prevent the injury. So, stability ability does that keeping. Therefore, to prevent injuries stability training of upcoming action or sport should be done.

Creating better force is related with stability as well; not the stability of moving joints' but those of not moving joints of limbs. For example, a baseball thrower doesn't need any stability in his arm or shoulder for that particular movement of throwing. However, he needs to be stabilized on the ankle-knee-hips and abs chain to take force from the ground without losing the force on the way. Most of the sports requires this stability even those which sportsmen not touching the ground in it. Swimming for example, requires abs stability due to not lose the gained force through strokes, to make horizontal waves in water. Professional swimmers move like bullets, by contracting their abs all the time. It should be in this way. Otherwise they would lose too much momentum. This kind of stability is a summation of many joint's stabilities.

Best way to increase stability is working out with isometric exercises.

3. Strength

As muscles grow and get stronger, nerves grow and get stronger too. They get big in order to transfer many electrical waves at once so they can stimulate whole muscle more effectively. They get stronger, by creating more conjunctions; in order to transfer the stimulation faster. These physiological developments cannot be seen by eye from outside. But it can be felt during action.

Possessed amount of muscle is not important if you are not able to contract and use them. For example, there are bodybuilders who have got enormous legs, but they hardly can jump. However, a regular basketball player can jump a few times more than them. Even if their total weight is same. Because that basketballer is jumping for over 10 years. All day and every day. He has got muscles but more importantly nerves know how to contract them how to use them. Also knows to do that in very fast way. Same thing applies for bodybuilder in squat movement. Performing that particular movement probably for many years and showing more strength in that compared to basketball player, even if their leg muscle mass is same.

A contraction we see as one actually is, hundreds of contractions in muscle. For example, while a sedentary person can contract his leg muscles while jumping for 10times in a second and we see summation all of those contractions as one weak movement. A professional basketball player can contract his leg muscles while jumping for 100times in a second and we see summation all of those contractions as one strong movement. The contraction number difference; between educated muscle and uneducated is may be close to these numbers. These numbers are very special and different for every person and for every movement. It is the muscle-nerve education that decides to these numbers.

Most common example to these adaptation and development is difference with dominant hand and the other hand which feels like it belongs to somebody else for most people. Even though both hands' muscle mass is almost same. But ability of using those muscles, so the effectiveness of nerves; is different. That difference makes the dominant hand many times stronger in the terms of grip strength and being effective on skills.

Strength training is a must in order to create more force, create bigger moves at once. It is the third step of whole development, but always should be worked out for the ones who need it. As mentioned before, it is a lifelong skill and can be improved always, nobody is able to see their maximum limits because of limited lifetime. But many people made impressive things, a ton of punches or 40 inches of jumps and so on. All of these are related with improved strength ability of using muscles more effectively. The ones who show these achievements are most famous people of their sports and not most muscular people in their sports. However, they still may still show these achievements with that optimal muscle mass because of strength factor.

4. Hypertrophy

Hypertrophy is the word which basically explains growing of muscles. Training muscles doesn't mean they are always going to grow. Because growing is only occurring when it is necessary like all other improvements of body. By the mean of growing, we intend that muscle will get larger as volume. Due to increasement in sarcoplasm, muscle requires much more core cells in order to manage the cell. So, by getting larger not only sarcoplasm increases; but, number of core cells, amount of ATP-CP storages and other related organelles increase.

This growing cost a lot to body, because bigger muscles are spending much more energy than smaller ones, even they never do actions. Because there is basal metabolism to make them continue to their existence. 1 Kilogram of muscle normally burns out approximately 3KCal per hour in base level. Brain doesn't like this idea. Because brain always after increasing the survivability. However, burning more calories will make person need much more food, and when person is not able to find calories, it is going to run out of energy; so, in the long term, dying may occur much faster in this proposition of body. In the modern world dying because of hunger is not an issue to those who are wealthy enough to read these sentences. But brain doesn't count on this one. Still, there is one thing we can understand from these statements. The person with bigger muscles should eat much more calories to maintain his fat tissue and glycogen storages. On the other hand, we can think like this; a person who has got bigger muscles can burn out fat tissue much faster.

Muscles are force power of the body. Fibers of muscles don't increase in numbers, but their volume increases which we call as hypertrophy. Increased; volume, increased usage of ATP-CP/per second, increased ability of contracting much more volume; are bringing much more power. By the means of power, it is the force that can be created at once. That is why; people who is related with power sports are trying to get bigger muscles.

While considering sports performance, getting bigger muscles are not always good even for the person who needs force power. A common example; basketball players. They want to jump as much as they can, but if they increase their muscle volume more than a limit which is determined according to their Force/Weight ratio, it will make them jump lesser than they could. Because muscle is a source of power but at the same time a source of weight which is limiting the effect of power; which is movement. So, there is always an optimum limit of hypertrophy for; every power required movement which also related with this ratio. However, it is needed to be calculated specifically for every person. Making calculation for every person individually for every specific movement is very hard or impossible in today's possibilities. But generally professional coaches having an eye-calculation with the experience in the field, also sportsmen may feel it in long term.

5. Power

It is a term which is related both with strength and hypertrophy. That is why it is the 5th step of the ladder. Hypertrophy is the source in order to create force, there is a direct relation between muscle volume and maximal power.

Having too much muscle mass doesn't always mean that person will have good maximal power or maximal force or "bursting power" in other saying. Because strength training is a must to educate muscle thus create excessive power. Getting muscle volume may be done by fitness or other sports with help of some equipment. Such as Leg Press Machine, a common example. However, by maximal power it is referred that; one rep squats which power lifters do or incredible jumps like professional basketball players do. Having muscles doesn't mean you can use %100 of them as you wish and when you want. Contracting them is bounded to ability of your brain and nerves. So, strength trainings are necessary in order to contract every muscle type and each fiber of those types in to reach and develop maximal power.

How strength training can be performed question has got a simple answer. With the same movement as you wish to show maximal power in it. If you want to jump higher, you have to make jump exercises with different variations. It is not meant that only and always performing jump exercises will make you to see your best limits. It will make you better, that is true but to make a person reach its maximum jumping limit there has to be perfect mix of hypertrophy training and strength trainings which conditioning trainers are expert on that. Power is not meant for daily usage or for normal people. It has to be acquired only by sportsmen. That is why it is the hardest and last step of the ladder.

Exercise science is still being improved so we may never see the perfect form of a person probably right now, but we may see most of the capacity that human may reach in todays condition in people; who are the best in their sports or in their fields. We watch those people in Olympics or in the best leagues which is specific for their sports.

Basic abstraction is of whole topic is;

Strength x Hypertrophy = Maximal power (power).

Chapter 3:

Exercise

Exercise Planning: Why and How to Exercise?

The reason of learning the exercise science, actually is; being able to answer the following questions and plan a proper exercise system individually;

1) Why a person should exercise?
2) What is the reason of to start exercising?
3) What abilities and physical improvements should have to be acquired according to that reason?
4) Which path has to be followed through this aim?
5) How do we know that, have we reached our aim?

First of all, it has to be known that; exercise is based on person and custom to person.

It has to be clarified as detailed; what person wants and how person is going to acquire it. It has to be considered as both physically and mentally.

Mentally it is being done by basic questions and if it is a person who wants to get improvement in any sports; then this mentality has to be put into a form of exercise to serve its desire.

Consideration all of physical attributes of person is more challenging than mental examination, and more required for planning and deciding exercises and it has got sub-steps which all have to be identified.

1.) Weight, Height
2.) Age
3.) Gender
4.) Sportive Background
5.) Current Muscle-Fat Ratio
6.) Past Disabilities and Current Disabilities

1.) Weight, Height

Weight is a keystone for every exercise program. It does decide every single element and exercise of the program. If person is over-weighted, that person have to stay away from athletic and plyometric exercises until he become eligible to do them as safely and properly. Because, overweight person would not be able to complete some of advanced exercises or would have injury risk while performing them.

If person under-weighted person most of the exercises will be proper for him. Still, heavy weighted ones like squat with weights may be unexpectedly failed in first repetitions. So, before start to exercise or select it, examining and trying with lower weights or forces; would prevent injuries. Starting from lesser load and increasing step by step is the safest way for anybody who is willing to exercise. It has to be done in this way while experiencing new exercises despite of our ego.

2.) Age

Age is a cornerstone. Human body changes with age more than we could foresee. Until entering puberty, creating muscle tissue and ability to create big forces are very limited.

It is a simple biology information. People who are living closer to Ecuador enter puberty earlier. And who are close to pole's are enter puberty later. The age values that we will talk on; generally, are based on European latitudes. It always should be considered for every person individually.

In last phases of puberty, a person has too much energy, but creating big force is still limited. A person who is between its 16-20 (Depending on ethnic origin) has too much endurance when you compare last phase of adultism.

After puberty, so again changing with ethnic origin, between 20 and 25 ages, people find a balance between endurance and power. For athletic sports, these ages are most effective ages in the field. But depends on required physical contact. Sports such as basketball, having endurance could not be the most important thing.

Power is not always to force others. Power is also being used to force ground as well. So, jumping higher and running faster are also related with power.

After 30 years old, person loses its endurance when compared to younger ages but becomes to its most powerful form. In the terms of muscle mass and force create, person living its gold ages in these ages. An athlete or a sedentary person much be powerful but cannot perform his athletic skills in long durations compared to younger ages. It has a relation between increased muscle mass and increased total mass as well. Because increased muscle mass and total makes, lower endurance due to excessive energy source usage and metabolic waste creation. Even though these are not increased, body's regeneration gets lower.

As poet Dante said, 35 is the half of the way. At least for the human physiology. Because after 35, everything starting to go back. Endurance, muscle mass, force creation. But this does not mean that a person cannot make progress after 35. For someone who has not attended to sports or who didn't see its maximum limits yet; still could make a progress. 35 is a limit for a person to see maximum limits of its body. If he did not acquire maximum limits until that age, he will never see its body's best. If he starts after 25 or 30's to the activities, he still may see good results, but he could have been better if he started earlier or try its best earlier.

Longer explanation; For example, an athletic sportsman as a footballer or a basketball player or a similar sportsman is not able to be better after his 35's again depending on ethnic origin. It might be 31 or 39. So it is the reason many of the players retire in their 35 or 36. They are feeling that; they are going back, not being able to play better as before. Even they make insane workouts, body starts to fall back.

As It is mentioned, that is because they are already in their maximum limits. So, they are feeling that physiological changing much more than a regular person.

In regular people who are called sedentary; even could start to any sportive activity in its 70's or 80's and still could make progress as physiologically. Because they are not even close their limits even for their age. A person's limits are extraordinary even though its age is high.

As abstract, 35 is a limit for who is aiming for top leagues. Because they are the best of the best. Even a person which shows %90 of body's limit, he may not be able to stay in that league. But in lower leagues, in any sport, you could see people who are 40-45 years old and still doing good job. Because their %90 of body's performance -scaling their whole lifetime- may be enough for those leagues.

A sedentary person or a normal athlete could still make a progress and still continue to extend his maximum's after 35; but with every age maximum limit is going down. That is why, people with high age cannot show high athletic capacity; and that capacity is going lower with every year after 35.

For a clear explanation with an example; Most famous running athlete, a male who has ethnic origin of black and lived in Africa during his childhood; and holding many world records for short distance running.

His Degrees for 100Meter Run;

Age 21: 10.03s

Age 22: 9.69s

Age 23: 9.58s

Age 24: 9.82s

Age 31: 9.95s (And he finished his career after becoming tenth of the race)

As it could be seen, he has seen his best in early phase of adultism. Late phase of adultism has been worst (except very young age.).

Due to his ethnic origin probably, he entered his puberty while 10-11 years old. So normally as we said 35 years old turning back phase; becomes 30-31 years old for him. Because he entered puberty earlier and seen his limits earlier than people who born in mid latitudes.

If he would continue to run formally. Probably he would see this results in 100meter;

Age 35: 10.03s

Age 40: 10.75s

Age 50: 12.85s

Age 60: 13.45s

Age 70: 15.80s

But even in age of 70, he would still be able to see 15.80s. As it could be seen, human limits are extraordinary even though its age. However, we have calculated maximum limits though on a person who dedicated his life to that sport.

That means any human might continue to make progress until see these kinds of results, in any sports, with the same scaling.

However, expecting to obtain results of 60 years training in a few years; who has started to sport in 60's; is nonsense. We said that, person could continue to make progress but won't be able to reach these numbers. Also, his progress will be slower, compared to 20 years old person.

Everybody part slows as physiologically after 35. So, learning new information and new skills are slowing; because, brain physiology is slowing; Progress of power and endurance would be slow down as well, because of metabolism is slowing. But we should not break our courage with that.

Because everybody has to do their best for their condition, even though they started to sport in their late ages. Everybody has lack of something. For aged person it could be metabolism limits and progression speed. For younger person it could be the desire to stay health. It is better to have lesser physiologic limits than lesser desire. Because nobody can make any progress as physiologically without performing any exercise.

After many enlightening information about impact of age, we may say that. While deciding person's aim and deciding how to reach that, age is a cornerstone to consider.

3.) Gender

Health science discovered that, gender effects many things. Everybody is prone to some conditions according to their gender. It could be a disease or in contrary a better physical feature.

It could easily be said that; in human genders; A male is able to acquire better exercise achievements and exercise capacity than a female; because of hormones and physical attributes. However, we are talking about maximum limits and that depends on many other conditions.

When we are aiming an exercise, we have to consider; the wanted results by person according to its gender too. As example in bodybuilding and fitness sports; females focused on different muscles and strength of different movements when compared to males. I am not saying that it should be in this way or not, but generally it happens in this way. So, we have to consider our aim according to gender's desires. It is the mental part.

In athletic sports; male and female classifications are competing apart from each other. The reason of that is physiological limit difference between genders. Normally, a high degreed athletic male always has to be stronger in his sport when compared to the high degreed athletic female in the same sports.

According to a scientific study; Females have 37-68% of muscle strength of males in general calculation.

While working out or making assumptions, we have to consider this cult. However, as it is mentioned before, there are many conditions those; this topic depends on. For example; a 25 years old woman, might be stronger than 15 years old male. Female with 5 years workout might be stronger than male without workout background, in the same age. There will be many conditions that we have to consider which will be mentioned too.

4.) Sportive Background

Sportive Background has to be examined very well, before aiming the exercise type and method. Because, long years of sportive background no matter in which athletic sport; leads to many differentiates when compared to sedentary person.

Even though, that person might had done it long time ago, still would carry its benefits in its body.

For example, better cardiac capacity and vascular system capacity which are too important for any athletic sport. Which are also the main factor of endurance as well. A person who had swum in his teen ages for a few years would have much more endurance capacity than who had not when compared in their 40's.

A person who had wrestled for three years would be much stronger than any sedentary person.

People may be tended and eligible to some exercises even they have never done before because of their sportive background.

So, while aiming our exercises and deciding them, we have to consider sportive background.

Is it enough to just ask which sports the person have been into? A person's answer may lead us wrongly. Because we could never know that; how much time he spent in trainings or skipped how many. Did he just observe or really had been a good athlete? Probably the answer will be better than how person had been.

We always should evaluate the situation in an objective way as much as possible. Thus, Objective Evaluation Methods should be used for further information and more correct information.

Objective Evaluation Methods

Heart Rate (Resting Heart Rate Monitoring)

Muscle Strength (Strength tests or just try with weights)

Endurance (Running tests for distances, 5K – 10K)

Agility (T agility test and similar tests which are specific to sports)

Postural Analysis (Static and Dynamic)

5.) Current Muscle-Fat Ratio

As it is mentioned in "weight" title; either low or high weights may prevent us doing some kind of exercises. It has to be considered that; a person with high weight may have high muscle percentage in total body mass. That means that person should not be qualified as not being able to make some movements. And a low weighted person may be carrying too much muscle than we expected.

With a muscled person and sedentary person; there is not that much muscle weight difference. Actually, there is if you try to gain, but in weighting scale; additional 10 kg muscle of 70 total weight, doesn't mean that much of a burden when it becomes to performing exercise. A person may have very less amount of muscle and could be 70 kilograms while a person with enormous amount of muscle may be 70 kilograms as well. The main point on weight consideration is the muscle-fat ratio, not the weight's itself; henceforth the ability to perform activities.

A muscular male approximately has got 40 or 50 percent muscle mass in his body. It drops in female to 30 to 40 percent. And on a sedentary person that is around of; 30 – 40 for male and 20 – 30 for female.

These values are mean values. They might be lower or higher we always have to consider that. Because there will be always people with extreme values for both sides.

On the side of Fat;

- 0-10 Percent fat is low 10-20 normal and 20-30 is high for males.
- 0-15 percent fat is low, 15-25 normal and 25-35 is high for females.

These values are being used by health authorities. But in sports, those have to be considered; ethnic origin, age, aim of the person, current sportive aim. For example; a boxer might want to be in normal range of fat ratio; while fitness model wants to go lowest on fat, as much as she or he could, when going on a podium.

6 percent fat might be optimum for a fitness model or a soccer player; but it is too low for a rugby defender or a boxer. The "normal" changes on person.

The point of these information is to know normal expectations. In this way we could measure our values based on individual by comparing them with the normal values. However, planning an exercise and using all information is a complex job. That is what differs a specialist with the whole information in a book. A specialist knows many topics and cases about an issue; and bringing a solution by combining them. After completing this book, you will be learned all of these topics and become a great evaluator. But always you have to have this in your mind; you have to combine them and be open minded. An issue is always related to many topics; because we are talking about most complicated biological form; which is human.

A commonly used term; Body- Mass Index (BMI), which calculated by dividing your weight to your height. It is easy-to-use protocol but not accurate one. Because a fitness model may be calculated as underweight and a basketball player who plays in center may be calculated as obese in BMI. But in reality, we know that; it is being mistaken that results, because of people's: either their fat ratio is too low, or their muscle mass is too high; and those kinds of machines are usually created for sedentary people, in the light of mean data. This kind of districted calculation is not preferred in sports and exercises. Therefore, I am not sharing normal values for this index. Instead of that, I am sharing 6 steps of evaluation.

We always have to consider Muscle and Fat Ratio according to the age, gender, ethnic origin, aim, current being performed sport, sportive background, disabilities. In this way it could be considered that; If a person should lose fat or has to gain muscle or vice versa.

6.) Past Disabilities and Current Disabilities

Is there any kind of handicap on a person, is always has to be examined? A handicap may be weight, height, age etc. and it also may be a disability.

Every disability can be understood by evaluating and asking to the person. There are various disabilities; either gained from born or in life. It may be small or big.

A few examples;

A person who teared its anterior cruciate ligament which placed in knee. That person wants to start or continue some sportive activities. It has to be considered, is person gone through surgery and replaced ACL or not. If it is not replaced, we have to aware of loading pressure on knee may start hurting possibilities. Loading pressure in movements such as; squats, running and making zic-zacs while running. If it is replaced, new ligament level has to be examined and rehabilitative process of that ligament has to be considered in activities.

A person might have ruptured his infraspinatus muscle 20 years ago. He would compensate its absence in an abnormal way. We have to observe it and make our exercises according and along with that. "Normal" movement patterns cannot be forced to a person who lived with different functions for 20 years. That would not be helpful and if it is forced to make "normal" exercise or activity functions on that joint; probably another injury will show up. Because the body is not working as we know. A wrong movement for us may be a right movement for disabled person, according to his new body posture and neuromuscular system. Body adapts to everything. A person always has to be considered exclusively because of these adaptations before planning, evaluating and creating any exercise or activity.

If there is still no replacement of lost muscle or ligament which is common; we have to strength other enclosing muscles around that, to support that function. To take the burden of lost one, on their selves.

These were two examples of disabilities. One of them is occurred recently and other one occurred in the past. Including these two, there could be many forms of disabilities. Along with them, changes in the body functions and patterns. Correcting them or making activities and exercises with their presence is the meaning of expertise. It requires deep knowledge and case-based experience to get better.

Exercise Planning:

Isolated or Compound?

Which exercise cult is better? Is it isolated exercises or compounds? It depends on the person and on the aim.

Isolated

Isolate exercising has born with fitness and bodybuilding sports. In contrary of all other sports, most of bodybuilding and fitness exercises are aiming only size of the muscle, not the functionality in sports or in daily life. Ancestors of this sport have seen that focusing on one muscle group for a movement was way better than compound movements; for blood flow and oxygen usage for that particular muscle group. You were being able to lift much more weight with that muscle more than; you are loading on within the compound exercise. Because of much more circulation of blood and oxygen in that area, those can be spared for that particular muscle.

Our heart working with a pulse capacity depending on person. However, heart is not designed to feed all of the body with blood at the same time with %100 efficiency. If oxygen intake and blood flow is being shared with other muscles the weights that are being lifted will drop to lesser amounts on the activity of aimed muscle group.

With limited time, in order to get bigger, isolated exercise may be better choice.

Compound

With the years, people have developed new ways to train muscles for athletic sports. Which makes them be able to; run faster, turn quicker and use full body power more efficiently.

Athletic sports such as football, basketball and so on, requires these kinds of abilities. In this situation, working out in compound plan; would make these abilities improve, much more than isolated exercises; due to creating and improving a pattern of nerve stimulation which is the main source of strength. Only with the condition of working out with correct exercises.

In athletic sports, we are using many muscle groups in the same movement. For example; while making a body turn with the ball in any of these sports, a person is using;

-Quadriceps, Hamstring and Glute muscles for pelvis stabilization.

-Internal rotators of one leg and external rotators of other leg.

-Core muscles for Upper Body Stabilization.

-And arm muscles to balance the body in its new stance.

As it can be seen, any simple movement of an athlete includes very compound usage of muscles. Training muscles and movements in compound way will teach the muscles to being used in that way.

Muscles and nervous system have got a memory and ability to learn patterns. It is also why the dominant hand of a person works way better than the other hand; because person has made much more practice with the one since he born, and that hand learned many more patterns and how to make them more efficiently and faster.

There is one more benefit of compound exercises, which is time saving. If many muscle groups trained in one movement, which we call it "compound", working out many muscle groups in restricted time would be possible. So, everyone's workout time is limited with hours in the day and with the days in the week. Specially for those who are not professional athletes.

Also, there is a fact that; to get optimum results, every muscle has to be worked out once in every 72 hours; because it completes its development in 72 hours.

If it is aimed that; to be more athletic and save some time due to workout time restriction, compound exercises might be better for that person.

Choosing

"Do I have to choose one? Am I not able to be athletic and big sized at the same time?"

It is possible. Compound and isolated exercises may be mixed in a workout plan. I suggest that. Everyone's aim is different, you could want efficiency in some of your muscles while you want blasting power and size in some of them. Then mixing them in correct way would solve the issue.

For example; Basketball player trains mostly in compound way, but in order to jump higher and run faster they add a leg extension exercise with weights to their routine which is an isolated one. So, in this way they train their Quadriceps muscle with almost %100 efficiency by the means of hypertrophy, which make those muscles bigger and more powerful.

As abstract; Confirming the absoluteness of "one of them is better than the other" is impossible. It depends on the body and the aims. Everyone has to have a custom workout plan individually.

	Isolated	Compound
Pros (+)	Size	Athleticism
	Power	Time Saving
Cons (-)	Not Being Capable of Doing Effective Complex Movements.	Not Using %100 power During Exercise of the Active Muscles
	At least 4 Days Workout Routines to work out every group of muscles.	Small Sized Muscles, less bursting powered Muscles

Exercise Planning:

Exercise the Heart or Not?

One of the main components of designing an exercise is heart rate and heart performance. It is important for both; being aimed and being a limiting factor.

Improving heart capacity, dropping heart rate, improving cardiovascular health and capacity may be aimed, then which workout type better may be decided in the terms of intensity and intervals. One of other aims may be the first choice; then, cardiovascular capacity should not be a limiting factor. How to make it possible?

HIIT (High Intensity Interval Training)

HIIT (High Intensity Interval Training) is a method which originally developed from human nature and activities. This training or activity method requires to use most of the potential of body in one phase which is why we call as "High Intensity". Interval in the name stands for resting periods. These periods may be in the form of active resting, like still performing a kind of activity with some of potential of body; or may be in full resting form. Resting period should be in a limit to be still in same exercise and not to be separated. In this workout period, most of the potential of the body have to be used for some time. "Most of the potential of the body" refers to High Heart Rate numbers. Which can be vary for everybody. Even if it is described in percentages; it may differ with age, weight, gender. But there should be an objective to limit and that limit should be easy to understand; that, while working out, is the person in the HIIT or out not working out in HIIT protocol. If the exercise or activity performer can talk more than 3 words in one breath; that shows us, he is not using most of his potential. This limit works for everybody who from whichever variation. Because of; heart rate is limiting factor in this kind of training; heart performance is being improved significantly with this training. Because of adaptation rule of the body.

In order to not limit HIIT workout with; Type IIb muscle fibers' activation time, instead of Heart Rate; the muscle group which is being used may have changed with another muscle group during the activity phase, or the volume of usage may change between three grades. In this way, Type IIb muscle fibers may refill their storages while other type of muscle fibers or other muscle groups are being active and keeping heart rate relatively high.

HIT (High Intensity Training)

HIT (High Intensity Training) is the type: working out with most of the potential without giving any resting in training. By most of the potential, it is meant that, less potential than in HIIT. Because that won't be possible to use that much potential without resting. This kind of activity time is limited in human body no matter who we are talking about. Which is usually limited with Type IIa fibers' activation time. Because in this kind of workout, heart rate never sees its limits and it does not be a limiting factor.

Stabile Training

Stabile Training is working out in almost same condition for a long time. One example is, running for 10 Kilometers at once. It uses some of the potential of body which very far away from being most. But this training may continue for too long and without changes in the volume of activity. Limiting factor is neither heart nor muscle activity time in this one. Limiting factor is metabolic level of body, and this factor is very hard to improve.

Comparison

All of these training methods are mainly planned according with the Heart Performance Capacity. As indirectly these are related with muscle fiber types. Because;

* In HIIT, to increase the Heart Rate that much; Type 2b muscles and other two fiber types has to be used at the same time.

* In HIT, to keep the Heart Rate for that much time; Type 2a and Type I muscles has to be used.

* In Stabile Training, to keep Heart Rate low and to keep activity continuity that much; only Type I muscles has to be used.

To adjust heart rate level; and decide to "Is it going to be a limiting factor which has to be improved or not?" is based in muscle fibers' type activity. Because, besides basal metabolism activity, the only thing that uses heart's blood is muscle. Basal metabolism activity changes during the day with many parameters. However, muscle activity only occurs with movement, and different intensity of using muscles; changes kind of used muscle type activity. With increased intensity of movement, more than one of muscle types are being activated in the same muscle group, therefore much more blood is needed. That is the relation between muscle and heart.

Chapter 4:

Nutrition

What to Eat?

Eating is a must in order to perform activity of living. Furthermore, it is necessary in order to show a performance in activities. But what people should eat, and should everybody eat the same way has been two questions since the beginning of nutrition science.

Everybody is different and every-body is different so there are many parameters on what people should eat.

The age is an important parameter, because every age has got its own necessities. A growing baby, a toddler, a child has to take way more protein, minerals and calcium and so than an adult person; an adult person has got to take more than elders.

Gender is a parameter; protein intake of man has to be more than woman even they both are not making any exercises.

Body proportion, the fat-muscle ratio is important factor to consider. Two 100kg man, one of them with %10 Fat of total body weight and the other one with %35 Fat of total body weight; they should eat completely different to keep their ratio in this way. If they want to change it, nutrition is changing too. More muscle will require much more carbohydrate and fat to consume. Even without exercise, those additions of nutrition will be required for basal metabolism of the increased muscle mass and the internal organs which has increased their activities with increased muscle mass. To repair and keep alive muscle and internal organ cells, protein requirements increase as well. And, with presence of exercise that intake of protein-carbohydrate-fat gap, between non-exercising person, would enlarge.

Basal Metabolism Rate, it changes with age; but there is one factor that never be changed, which is genetics. Everybody starts to life with different basal metabolism rate, because everybody has got different kind of metabolism. Even muscle mass increased or decreased, age changed, or any other thing applied; some guides in the body never changes. Our muscle mass, height, weight, internal organ activity is limited by genes, henceforth our basal metabolism rate as well.

Activities and type of activities; different activities with different intensities and volumes are activating different kind of muscle systems, therefore the energy storage which is being used change. Because of that, body will be in a need of required nutrition which is special to that kind of muscle type activity.

What Human Should Eat?

Everybody should eat some nutrition according to body ingredient, their daily and sportive activities, age, gender, genetic branch, and special situation such as diseases.

Nutrition Types

Every nutrition has got different type of; digestion, storage, and usage. Always taking one of the nutrition's will end with malfunction of some systems in the body. Fat may be optional for this phrase, because body is able to turn carbohydrates to fat. But every nutrition is meant to do something so, even we are not taking fat, we will produce some fat in order to use that in the relevant actions. That is why there is a minimum healthy fat limit for every person. Because humans need it.

Carbohydrate is may not be considered necessary, but glycoses is. In order to create too much ATP in limited time it is necessary to have glycoses in the body. So, one way or other body is going to take glycoses and taking carbohydrates is easiest way to do that.

A) Fat

It is the kind of nutrition that has strong biochemical structure. Due to its structure it is very long to digest but at the end, it is giving the award of that struggle. 1 Grams of Fat contains almost 9Kcal which has no equal between energy sources. Then why we are not always taking fats and using them? Because it is not possible for human mouth taste and it is not effective as it is sound as.

Because, fat molecules are being broken in 6

minutes in the presence of oxygen. Without oxygen they don't break. Oxygen carriage capacity of blood is limited and some of the movements require ATP very rapidly. 6 minutes is a very, very long time for them; such as Brain activities or forcing muscle activities.

Fat is mostly used for internal organ activities and slow twitching muscle fiber activities which we usually use them in daily activities such as walking or writing on computer. Even if we don't do anything fat is being used in internal organs in every minute. Because they always create the basal metabolism. It is being used in these areas because, there is no ATP rush in these areas. ATP is being used over time and for long time. Fat digestion and breaking metabolism perfect design to use in these functions.

B) Carbohydrates

A gram of carbohydrate is equal almost 4Kcal energy in human body. It is being digested fast therefore; if it is not used in limited time, body decides to storage is as fat if additional is taken. By the additional it is meant, more than glycogen storages can take. A normal 70kg male holds around of 2000Kcal glycogen storages in their body, 1500 in muscles and 500 in liver. Body is able to hold that much of glycogen without using it in order to use in necessary actions. However, much more than that is not necessary for storages. Because these much glycogen can be enough of energy source for a non-sportsman person for around of 3 days. Usually in the modern world if a person is not an athlete, a person always walking around with filled storages. Therefore, every eaten food has to be turned into fat in order to store. Because body wants to make savings, not wasting.

Fast twitch actions which we know as sprint or weightlifting kind of activities and brain actions -which are pretty ATP consuming in a limited time- are using glycogen storages thus carbohydrate. It is necessary to take carbohydrates in order to keep their performance up. Otherwise, body is going into saving mode, because of its survival instincts and adaptative nature.

Body turns into saving mode, but also still uses glycoses. Henceforth it has to produce glycoses from somewhere, which is the long-term storages, so fat. Fat cells may turn into glycoses in the liver with the process of gluconeogenesis. It is a kind of turning that is healthy and normal, but if somebody is going through action which is not accorded with saving mode, such as athletic performance; this kind of creation will be still enough for to complete movement. However, body will not be in the will of giving the maximum performance; due to hardness of this process and uncertainty of future. Is this person going to take enough of fat or carbohydrate in following hours and days? Nobody knows and, body is trying to be always prepared to uncertainty.

C) Proteins

Everybody has got protein structure in their body; so, to keep that protein system active and continue to mitosis and repair in body; everybody even the old people has got to take protein every day. Why "everyday", will be explained in "When to Eat?" section.

Protein is not a source of energy but a source of building in the body. It is being digested in the requirement of anabolism in the body, which we know as growing, muscle creating, repairing. Other than those, body never takes proteins into blood flow in people, except who have sicknesses. Because there is nowhere to store proteins in the form of storage. Also, body is not able to create spare muscles or spare cells in order to use in further situations, with that additional protein. So, the excessive protein intake will always find its final form as uric acid in the urine. If it is not making final at there, we will be talking about sicknesses such as gout. Which is a kind of arthritis and occurred because of excessive amino acid in the blood stream.

While calculating daily calorie intake, and while calculating total calories of a product, proteins are being calculated as 1g/4Kcal. If it is being burned in calorimeter, that number is correct. But body does not consume proteins to use it as energy. So, all the proteins should be calculated as "0" in calorie intake. Either protein is used as construction or thrown away from the body.

Proteins should be calculated in another calculation type which is protein intake.

Amount of protein is decided again with many parameters, but age and gender are two major ones. Adult Male has got to take 1,0 grams of protein for each muscle kilograms in his body every day, while adult female has got to take 0,8 grams of protein. These numbers are shared in the light of many examinations and variations of people. Adult is a wide word to use and there are many genetic branches which are changing these numbers. Even from the same genetic tree, two people may have another kind of metabolism than each other. So, these numbers are not restricted rules, but they are more likely a guide. Because these numbers are different and special for everyone. But there is one certain thing about protein intake; children and who are performing sports has to take increased protein than its non-sporting adult form in order to increase or keep their muscle mass. Old people who are generally accepted as more than 35 years old, may take less than their regular adult form intake in order to keep their body proportion as before.

D) Others

There are many kinds of minerals, vitamins and hormones, those have to be taken by human body from outside. Without their present in the body, some exiguousness symptoms start according to their function.

With the light of the researches, many of these "others" have been discovered and necessary amounts of them are enlightened. However, many of the "others" haven't even discovered yet, so we cannot talk about it. But we know that; they are not discovered yet, because the process of finding the current ones, took more than a century and we are still discovering new hormones etc. Most importantly, we still can't cure many diseases, which shows us we still lack information about human body.

1000mg of Calcium, 90mg of Vitamin C, 1.3mg of Vitamin B6, 600IU of Vitamin D... Everyday intake calculations and which may differ with age and gender... The main issue is; calculating them and trying to take them daily is impossible. Because there will be around of 40 pills and tons of food which not may be eaten in a day. Then "We have to let the body, do its job."

Body Doing Its Job

Body is a magnificent factory. Takes what is necessary and doesn't take what is not. Process in the right form what is taken. Store or use it in the right form. Always create "The Balance" and regulate everything.

Most of the people in the history, even never heard "Nutrition Science" and they have lived for more than 100 years. It is a necessary science but when it is required.

Eating; organic by growing and organic by processing foods and, eating them in a variation which is not selected by the desire, but by logic; is enough to take everything necessary. Not focusing on one food or nutrition and making a logical distribution according to genetics, age, gender, activity level would solve everything.

Even still if a person has got some sickness, some symptoms, some deficiency in the performance of activity, then the blood values may be examined. After examination, lacking nutrition will be given additionally or will be added to diet with foods and everything will be solved. Even, for wealthy enough countries or people; blood values can be examined regularly without any symptom or anything else.

That is the right path of "What to Eat".

When to Eat?

Isn't it all about, what to eat? Is timing important? Yes. Timing is important for two factors. One of them is general health and other one for athletic performance.

Eating is keystone of building the body and keeping that building as standing. However, eating is a reason of delay or deficient in the body as well. Eating starts a chain of process in the body which is really impactful. Too much calories are used during the process, many hormones pike in both ways, blood pump is used by digestion organs and many more.

It is inevitable to beware from these impactful changes in the body. But the wrong time is evitable.

What is the wrong time of eating? It depends on the ingredients of food. It will be explained but first; much more important question; why we beware from these impactful changes.

- Blood and oxygen and some of nutrition are being used for digesting. During the process, activity performance will get lower due to insufficient reach of rich blood to the muscle tissue.

- Hormone balances are in the sake of catabolism in order to catabolize the food in the belly. Two opposite hormones always balancing each other. During the presence of high catabolism hormones, anabolism hormones will get lower. Anabolism hormones are builder hormones of body. Insulin will increase and growth hormone will decrease during the digestion. Growth is a hormone which provide bigger muscles, bones and younger skin to us.

- With the increased insulin, the blood sugar levels will increase too. Frequently eating will keep blood sugar level and insulin level high. Due to adaptative mechanism of the body, a resistance of insulin will develop which is the main reason of Type 2 diabetes.

- Free fat acids in the blood -which are released to blood from digestion- will prevent releasing of leptin hormone. Leptin hormone is the main hormone which tear apart fat tissues and molecules. Frequently eating will decrease fat burning in the body and will be a reason to have fat which most of the people do not desire both for their appearance and health.

This far, it may be said that; eating frequently is not a good thing for health. Still some of the people may prefer to prioritize their athletic performance instead of health which is normal for professional sportsmen. However, that would be necessary only in a few rare cases.

"Do not eat frequently" that is okay. Is there a specific time to eat then?

Intervals of Eating

The perfect time for eating depends on everybody. Creating a universal fact is impossible. However, there are some scientific facts that should be used as a strong guide.

Most of the anabolism and regeneration occur during sleep. Entering to bed with full belly will sustain digestion during sleeping, therefore delay or defect of anabolism and regeneration will come up. "I didn't sleep well last night. I woke up tired." Entering to bed with full belly may be a reason. Even a person doesn't feel that kind of feeling when wake up, that doesn't change the result; that was not a sleep with quality. So, it is better to finish eating a few hours before sleeping for anabolism and regeneration of body.

How many hours exactly? Depends on the food.

Biochemical structure of proteins is too long to tear apart. Also, their physical bondage is too strong for stomach. They take many hours to digest. Meats may find 6-7 hours of digestion in the human body. Milk products around of 3-4 hours.

Fats are not that easy to digest as well. However, eating fats, may be a helper to eat less frequently. Because during digestion there will not be a feeling of hunger and they take really long to digestate. Also, fats are not increasing insulin level. Eating them during daytime may be a helper to the diet.

Carbohydrates are easiest to tear apart both physically and biochemically. They usually are digested around of 30min to 3 hours. 30 min for fruits, 3 hours for non-processed wheat products. Between these two there are tons of carbohydrates. Eating them to refill storages will be fastest way. If a person performs few times of high-level physical activities in one day, carbohydrates may be a good choice to eat during the day.

In exercise perspective, being eaten carbohydrates before exercise would affect performance positively. Having high level of glycoses and insulin in the blood giving body the expression of "you are not struggling with surviving; you can perform maximal effort of yours; we do not lack of food". Low level of insulin decreases exercise performance due to survival instincts. Because the person knows that; he is going to find food after exercise, but body doesn't know that and doesn't count on that.

Other than before sleeping meal, there are day meals or there is only one meal. That should be far away than the sleeping meal. Before sleeping meal, should be considered as the first meal. Second meal is the breakfast or if it is being skipped it is lunch then. Two meals diet is perfect for hormonal system, but exceptions may be made as mentioned before.

Body starts to anabolism and regeneration immediately after digestion stops. Growth and Leptin levels increase in the blood and everything going positively in the sake of health and getting fitter to the life. It goes in this way until eating and digestion starts over again. So, keeping this period as much as possible is good. But the limit is not infinity.

Body is thinking 24 Hours based. Going for same routine every day for 24 hours will make everything safer and much more adaptable.

Eating once in a day will significantly decrease energy usage of the body due to dipped down insulin level on the blood. It may be better for long living may be, not proven but who knows. But in proven science, it is not good for activity and brain performance. Eating twice in a day is perfect version for non-athlete people due to digestion time of the foods and the gap which has to be kept between first and second meals. Eating more than two meals only should be done in the presence of athletic performance or some special sicknesses.

Outroduction

There is no absolute perfect; living system, activity system, sleeping time, sleeping duration, exercise method, exercise duration and time, nutrition type, nutrition amount and time. There is no absolutism because every "body" and everybody is different. The book is meant to written in order to sharing essential information of the body in a solid way. Everybody has to make their custom "perfects". There is no trick or shortcut. Have a good luck at creating your "self-perfects".